The Art of Healing

A Glimpse of Cardiac Surgery

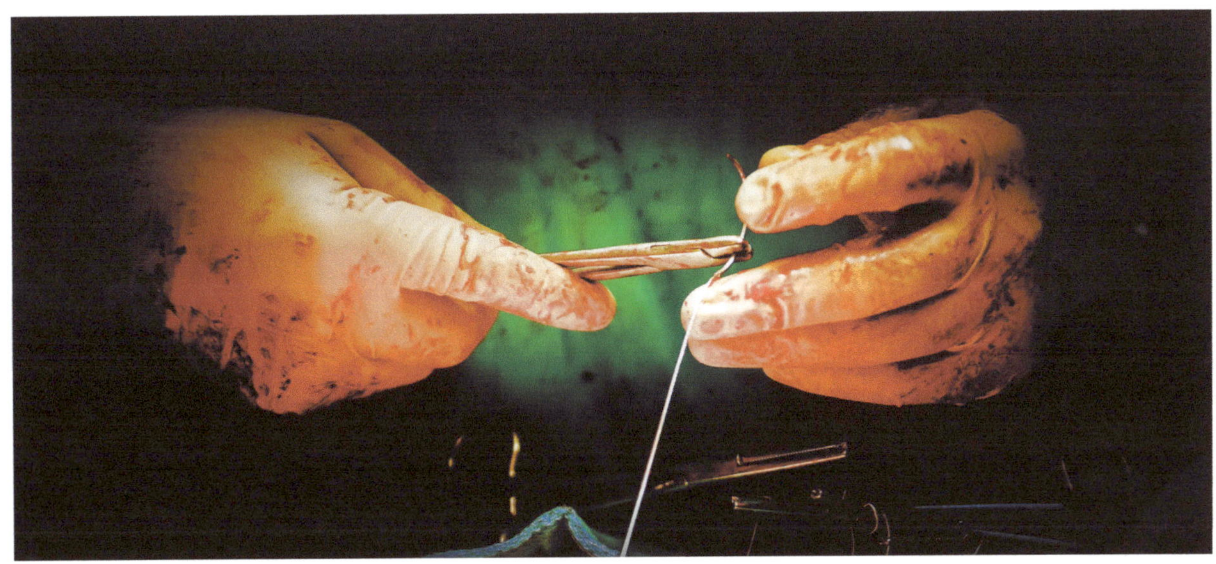

By **Ann Gilchrist**

With

Avinash Garg MD

ISBN: 978-1-9994676-0-9 (Paperback)

ISBN: 978-1-9994676-1-6 (Hardcover)

Submitted to the Library and Archives of Canada

The Art of Healing - A Glimpse of Cardiac Surgery

Published by Triple A Group

Email: tripleagroup283@gmail.com

Website: https://www.glimpseofcardiacsurgery.com

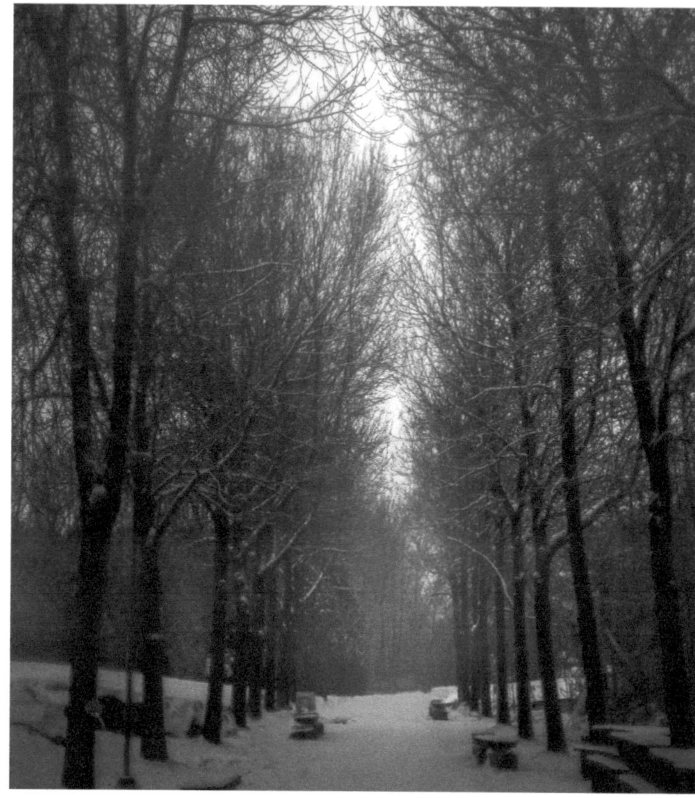

Science North Park, adjacent to Health Sciences North, Sudbury

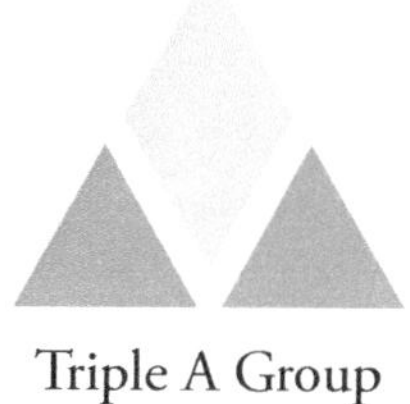

Triple A Group

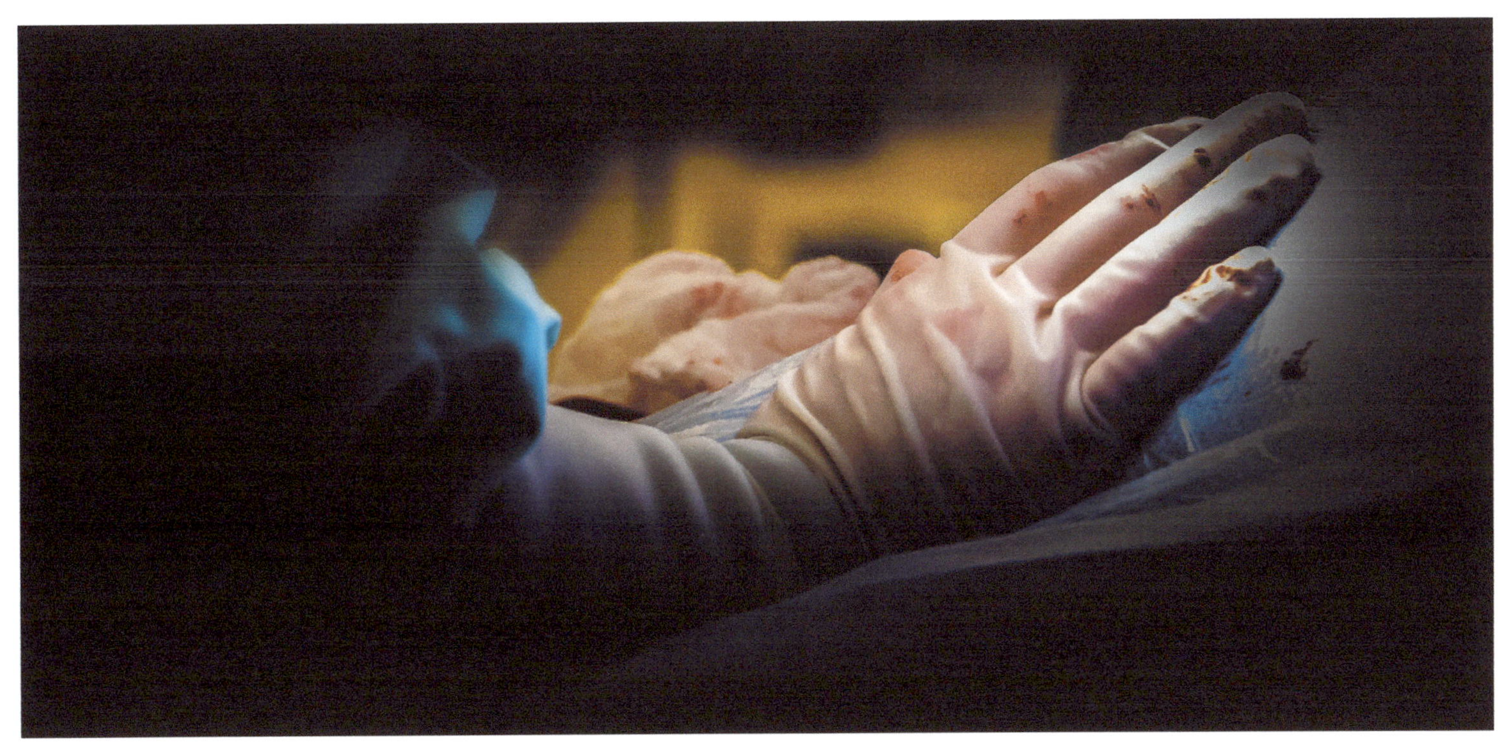

*Our sorrows and wounds are healed only when
we touch them with compassion*
— Buddha

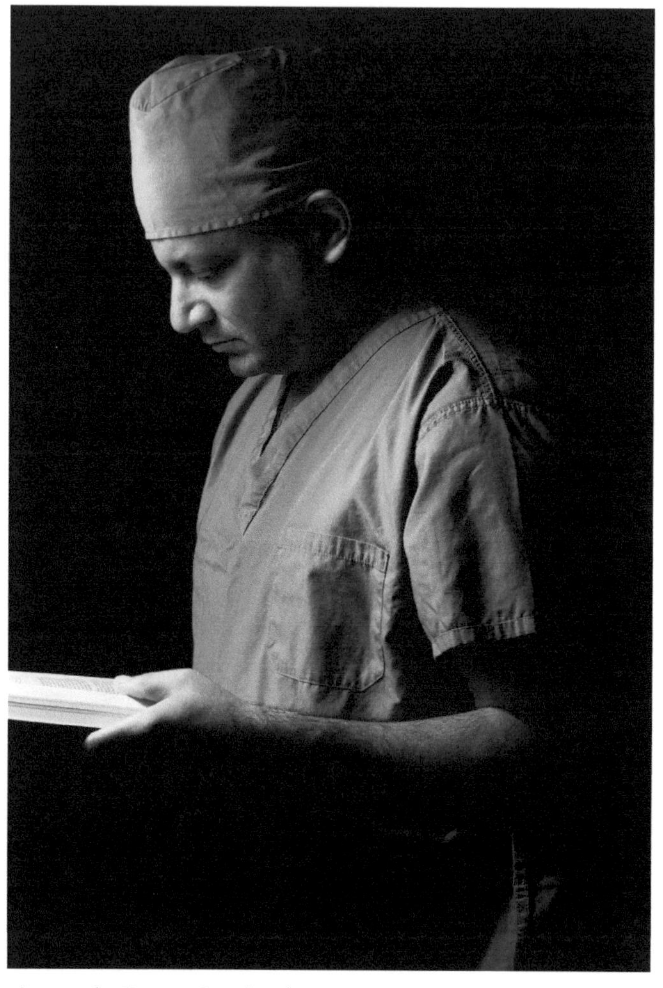

Avinash Garg, Cardiothoracic Surgeon

"Just like an artist who meticulously renders painterly solutions to compositional dilemmas creating an artwork cohesive in design, a cardiac surgeon artfully renders surgical solutions to complex issues of the heart, enabling the body to take over its healing process."
— Avinash Garg, MD

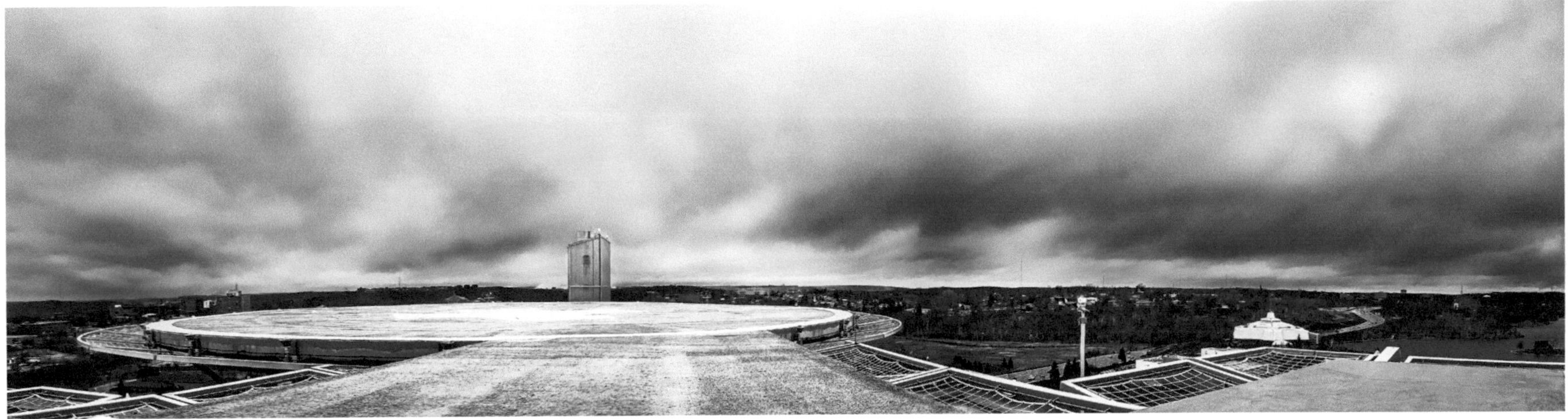

Helipad atop Health Sciences North, Sudbury, ON, Canada

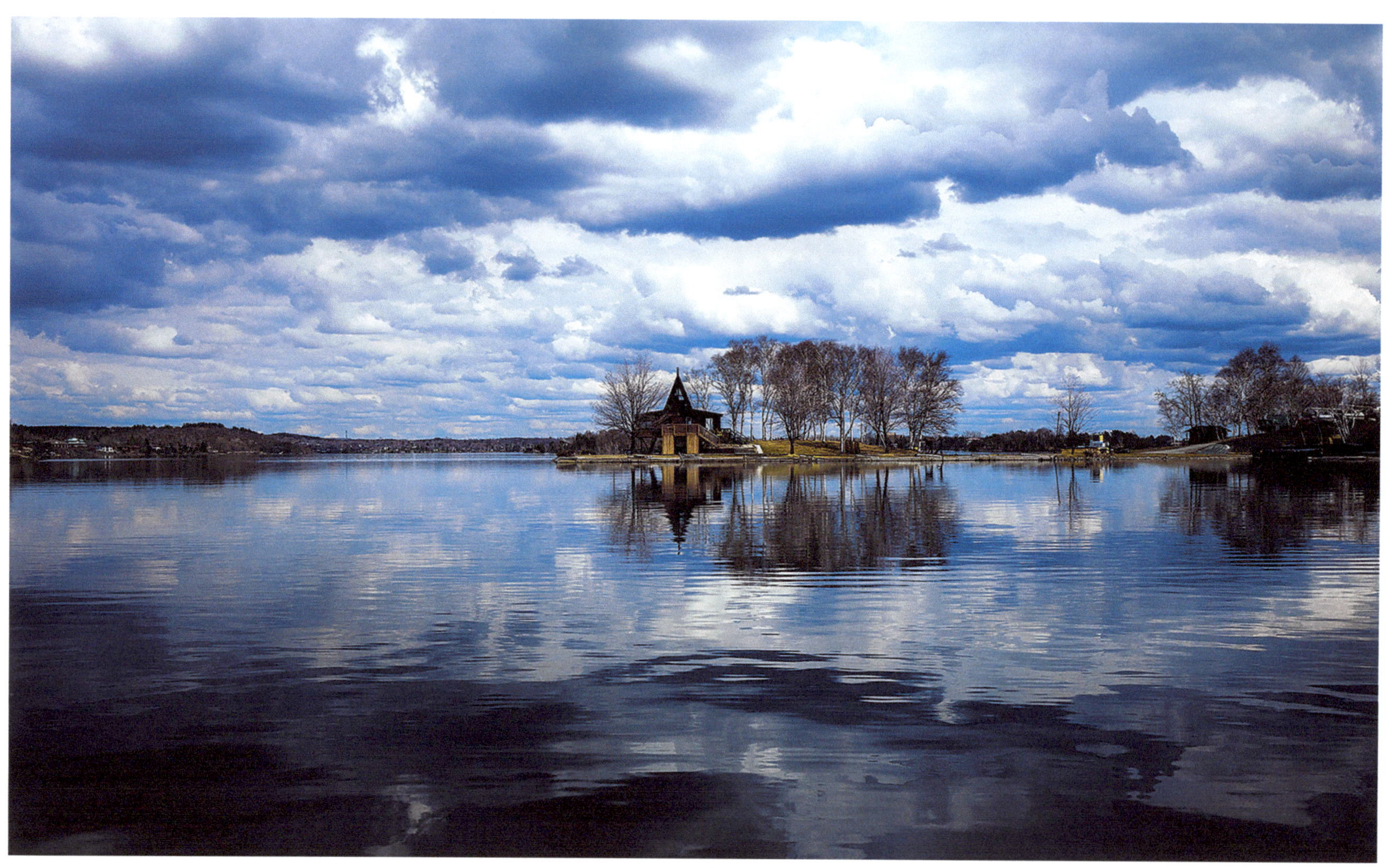

Sudbury, Ontario, Canada

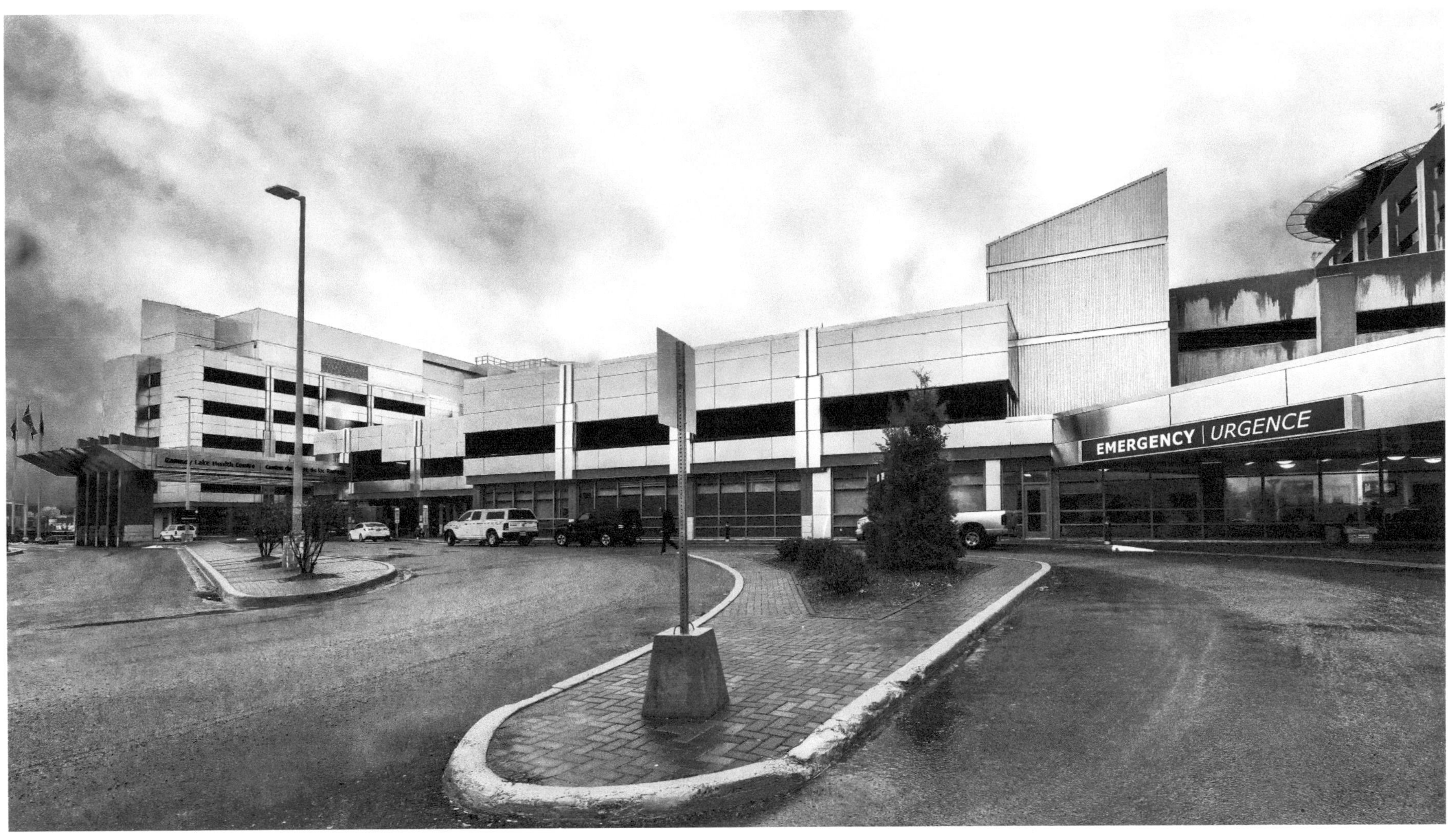

Health Sciences North, 41 Ramsey Lake Road, Sudbury, ON Canada P3E 5J1

My sincere thanks to the entire hospital administration and staff at Health Sciences
North in Sudbury for the opportunity to undertake this project.

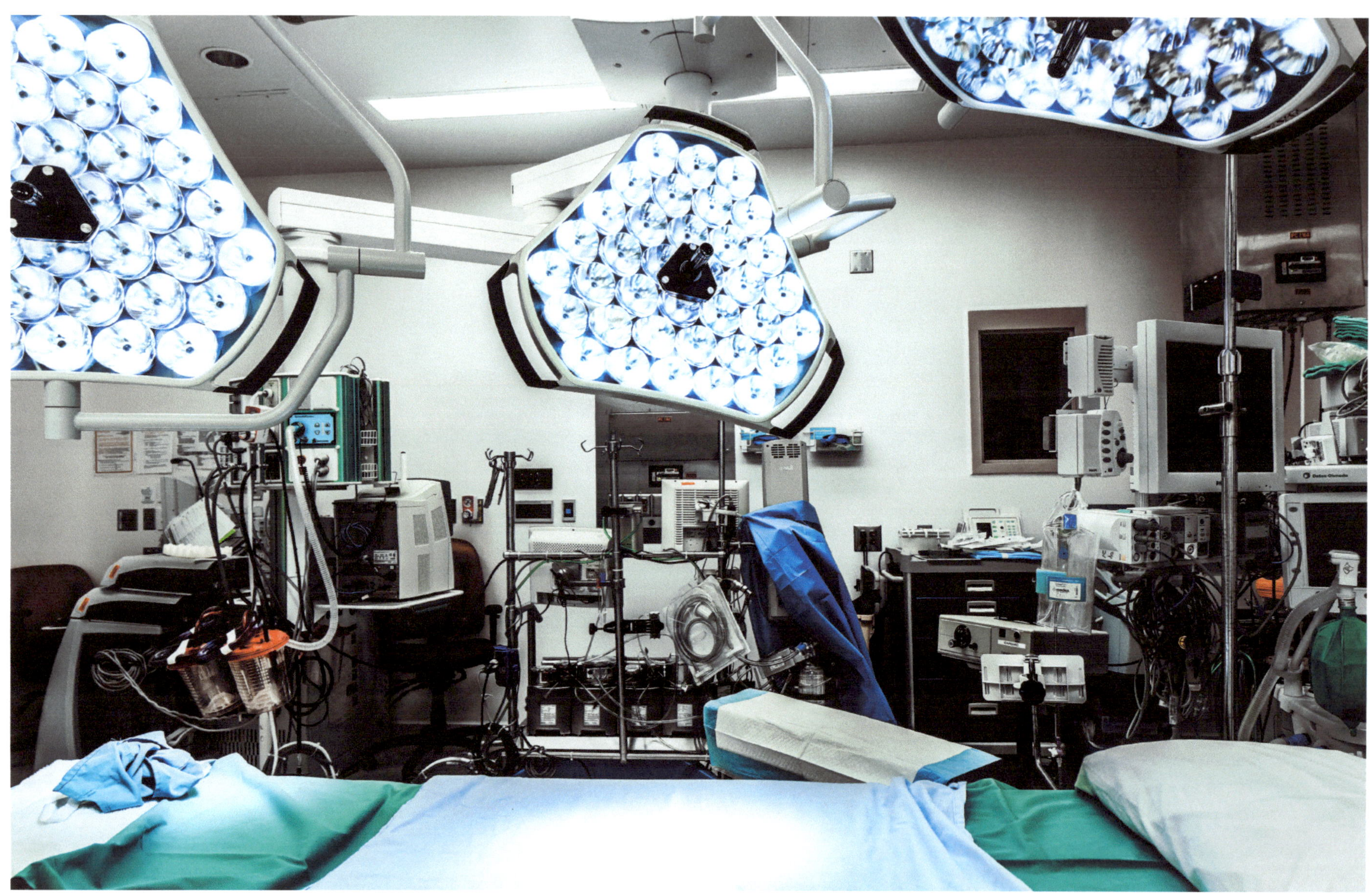

Operating Room 17

Contents

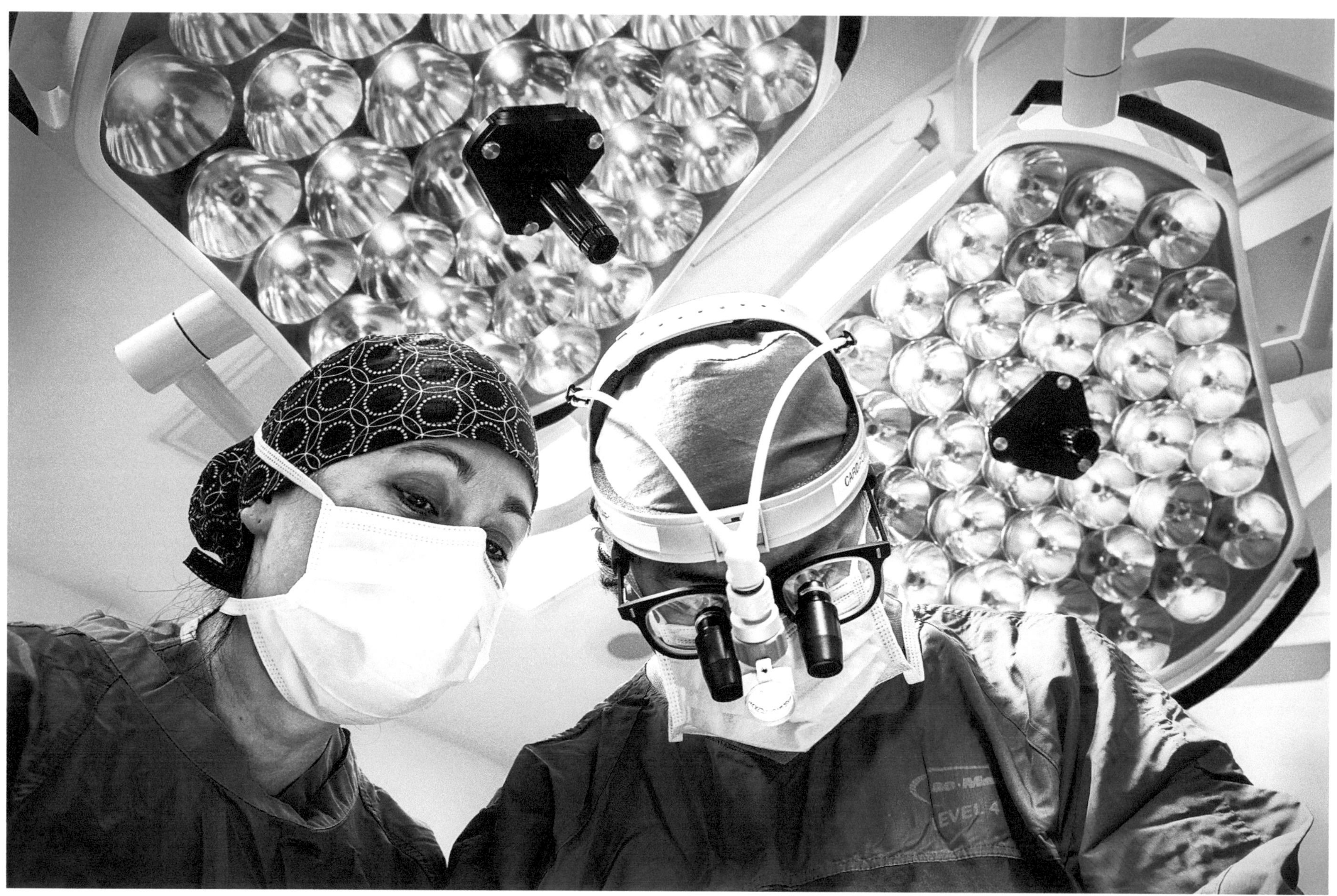

Avinash Garg, Cardiothoracic Surgeon, Operating Room Nurse Sandra Labrosse

PREFACE

This book offers a glimpse into a modern-day cardiac surgery operating room. Like virtuosos, the anesthetist, surgeons, perfusionists, and nurses execute an immensely complex procedure with impeccable harmony and precision.

Mastery in the operating room comes with a deep understanding of the discipline, with professionals enduring years of arduous academic training to meticulously hone their skills. Dr. Avinash Garg, the lead cardiac surgeon in these pages, grew up in Ottawa and attended the Ottawa University Medical School. He continued with post graduate surgical training at the University of Western Ontario to receive fellowships in General Surgery and Cardiothoracic Surgery from the Royal College of Physicians and Surgeons of Canada, in addition to a fellowship in Cardiac transplantation. Dr. Garg has been in clinical practice for the last twenty-four years.

I have worked for Dr. Garg in his office since he began his practice and have seen scores of anxious patients and families visit for pre-operative consultation. Apparent in most families visiting the clinic is the appreciable nervous tension about impending surgery of the family member, which usually stems from fear of the unknown. And so began the genesis of this book.

With a collection of photographs illustrating coronary artery bypass grafting surgery, this book reveals the workings behind modern operating room doors. My experience photographing the operation was sublime. The procedure was undoubtedly invasive, but I was struck by the commitment each person of the surgical team had in ensuring a successful operation. My intention was to document the entire procedure to explain the process of coronary artery bypass grafting in simple terms.

According to the Centre for Disease Control and Prevention, cardiac disease is the leading cause of death in North America. Many are affected by the disease or have lost a loved one to it. In my conversations with patients and their families, I found when they are clearly informed about the process, families are better prepared about what to expect, alleviating anxiety of the unknown. Long-term results following bypass surgery are outstanding, and patients feel immediate relief from their symptoms of chest pain. In fact, some patients notice a marked increase in their energy level following recovery and will quite often say they did not realize how much the disease had been slowing them down. It is truly remarkable how quickly most patients recover from the trauma of surgery. The patient followed in these pages was sitting upright in his bed twelve hours after the operation and was discharged from hospital five days after surgery.

I would like to express my gratitude to Dr. David Boyle, Medical Director of the Surgical Program, instrumental in making this project possible. Also, to Carol Kirkwood, Operating Room Manager, and Vivian Lapointe, Chief of HSN Communications.

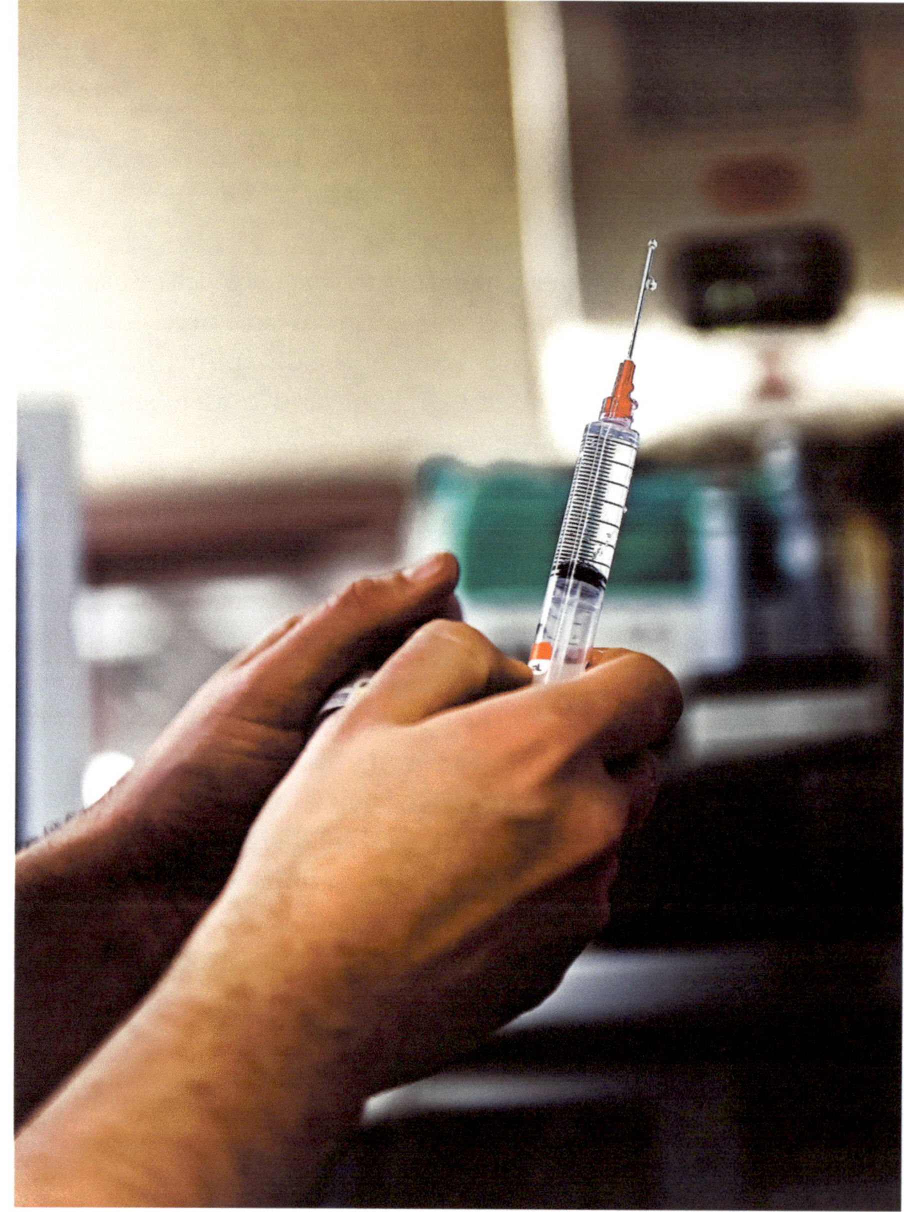

It all begins here

Anesthesia

Coronary artery bypass grafting, a highly complex procedure, involves multiple teams from various disciplines working closely together for the duration of the surgery, which is typically around five hours. They include cardiac surgery, anesthesia, cardiopulmonary perfusion, and the supporting operating room nursing staff. As a non-medical observer in the operating room, I was struck by the unison of each service, and from the moment I entered the operating room, orchestration of the surgical team seemed much like a string concerto at play—in perfect rhythm and harmony.

It all begins with anesthesia. The undoubtedly anxious patient is wheeled into the operating room on a bed where he meets with the doctors. Following a cordial introduction, the anesthetist and cardiac surgeon proceed with a patient checklist, where they formally identify the patient by name, the date of birth, operative procedure, and any drug allergies and communicable diseases the patient may have. Although the patient has been screened and has signed a written consent prior to entering the operating room, this is an added step in accordance with safety guidelines at the hospital. The background is bustling with nursing staff setting up instrumentation panels and equipment trays for the anesthetist. An electrocardiogram is attached to the patient to monitor cardiac rhythm. And, in a reassuring and comforting way, the anesthetist pulls up a stool beside the patient's arm, ready to insert various lines.

Perhaps at this point I will try to explain, in extremely simplistic terms, the anesthetic process. It is profoundly compelling to watch the patient drift into deep slumber, a state deeper than sleep, whereby the body loses its muscle contractility and its capacity to breathe on its own. Therefore, an external ventilator is required to breathe for the patient. The complex anesthetic process occurs in stages and involves monitoring, induction and maintenance of anesthesia, intubation and ventilation, and finally the reversing process whereby the patient is gradually eased back into consciousness once the surgical procedure is complete.

Anesthesia begins with the insertion of peripheral venous lines by way of catheters in the patient's forearm vein in the wrist, and in the median cubital vein in the elbow pit. The venous lines are primarily used for infusion of drugs. Once in place, the anesthetist proceeds with insertion of the arterial line in the patient's radial artery, in the wrist. The arterial line, connected to a device, is used to monitor the patient's pulse and blood pressure throughout the process. It is not uncommon for the physician to sometimes use ultrasound guided insertion of the arterial line in situations when tactile discovery of the artery on the patient's wrist is unsuccessful.

Sedation begins. Sedatives injected through the peripheral venous line, allow the patient to enter a relaxed or light sleep state, with drugs such as midazolam and sufentanil. The patient progresses into deeper sleep with the administration of intravenous anesthetic propofol.

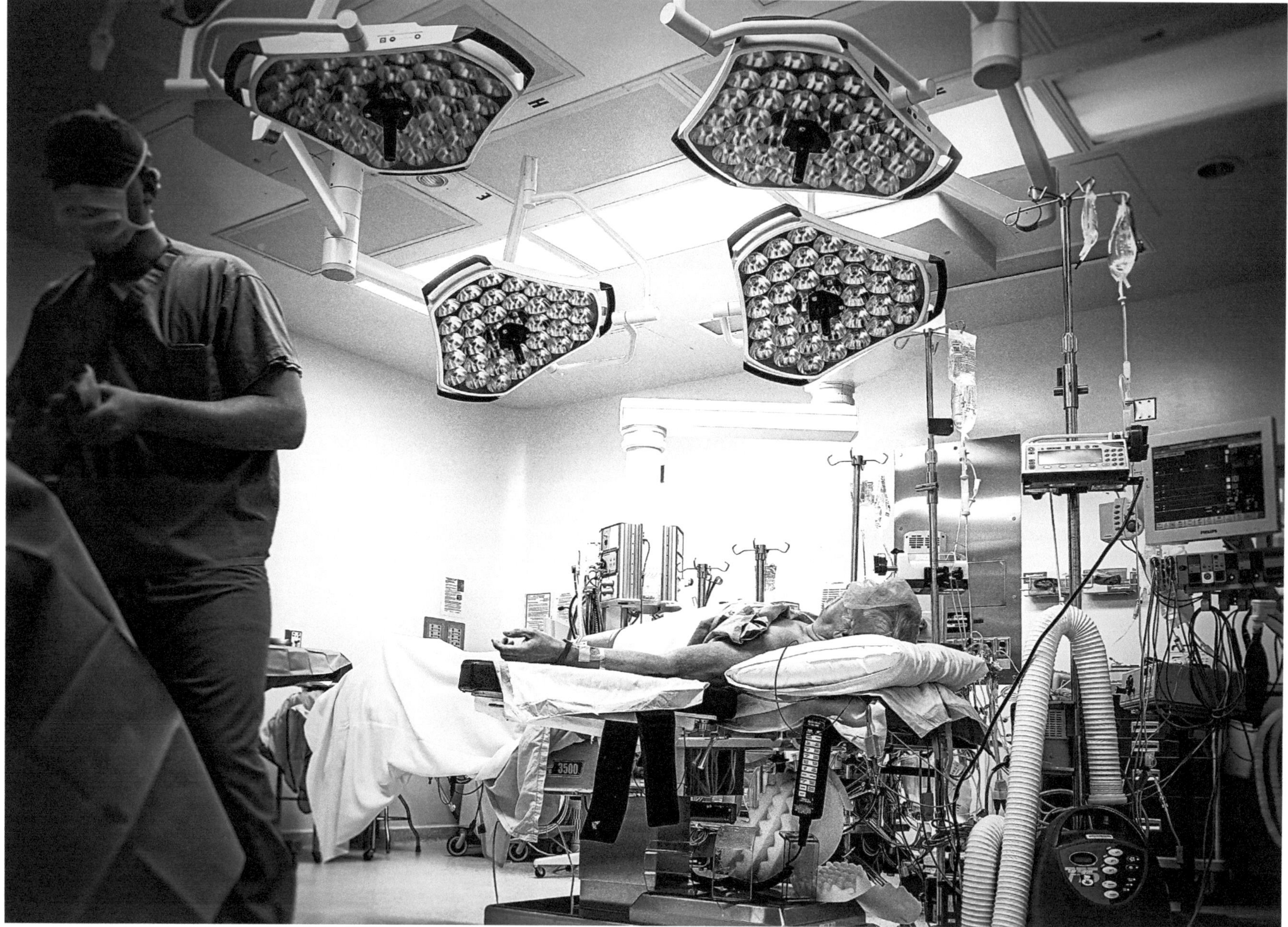

Patient wheeled into Operating Room 17

While drifting to sleep, the body also loses its innate ability to breathe with the administration of rocuronium, a muscle relaxant. The patient is pushed further into a deep sleep state with the administration of a volatile gaseous anesthetic, sevoflurane.

This was perhaps the most profound moment for me, as I watched the patient respond to these powerful medications. Within a matter of seconds, the patient drifted into deep sleep. Then, the anesthetist proceeded to insert a breathing tube in the patient's wind pipe connecting the ventilator to the patient, enabling external mechanical breathing, as the body's muscles are now incapacitated. I should point out that at this stage, muscle incapacitation does not affect the cardiac muscle, so that the heart continues to beat in rhythm.

With the patient soundly asleep, tracheal tube inserted, the anesthetist was gowned, and he proceeded to drape the patient in preparation for inserting the central venous line by way of the patient's jugular vein in the neck. The central venous line, in the body's larger jugular vein, is necessary for administering large volumes of fluid, medications, and monitoring central venous pressures as the procedure gets under way.

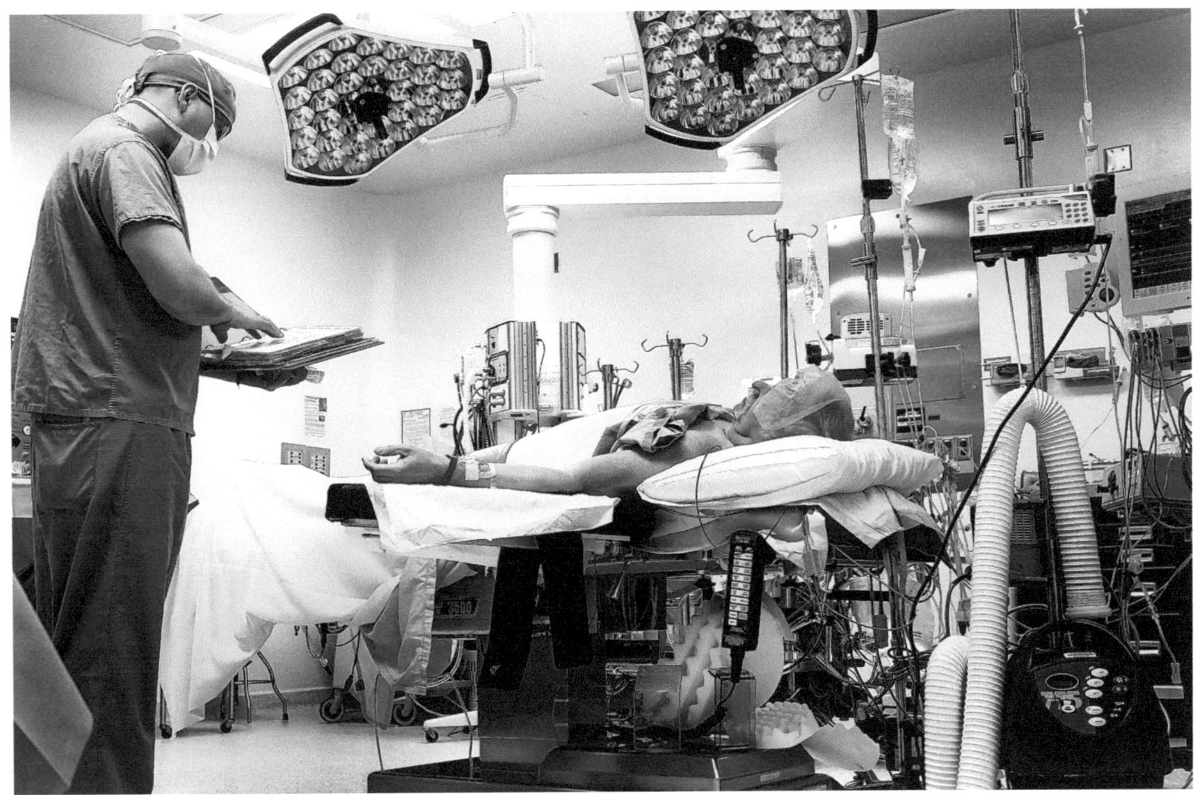

Patient identification checklist with anesthetist

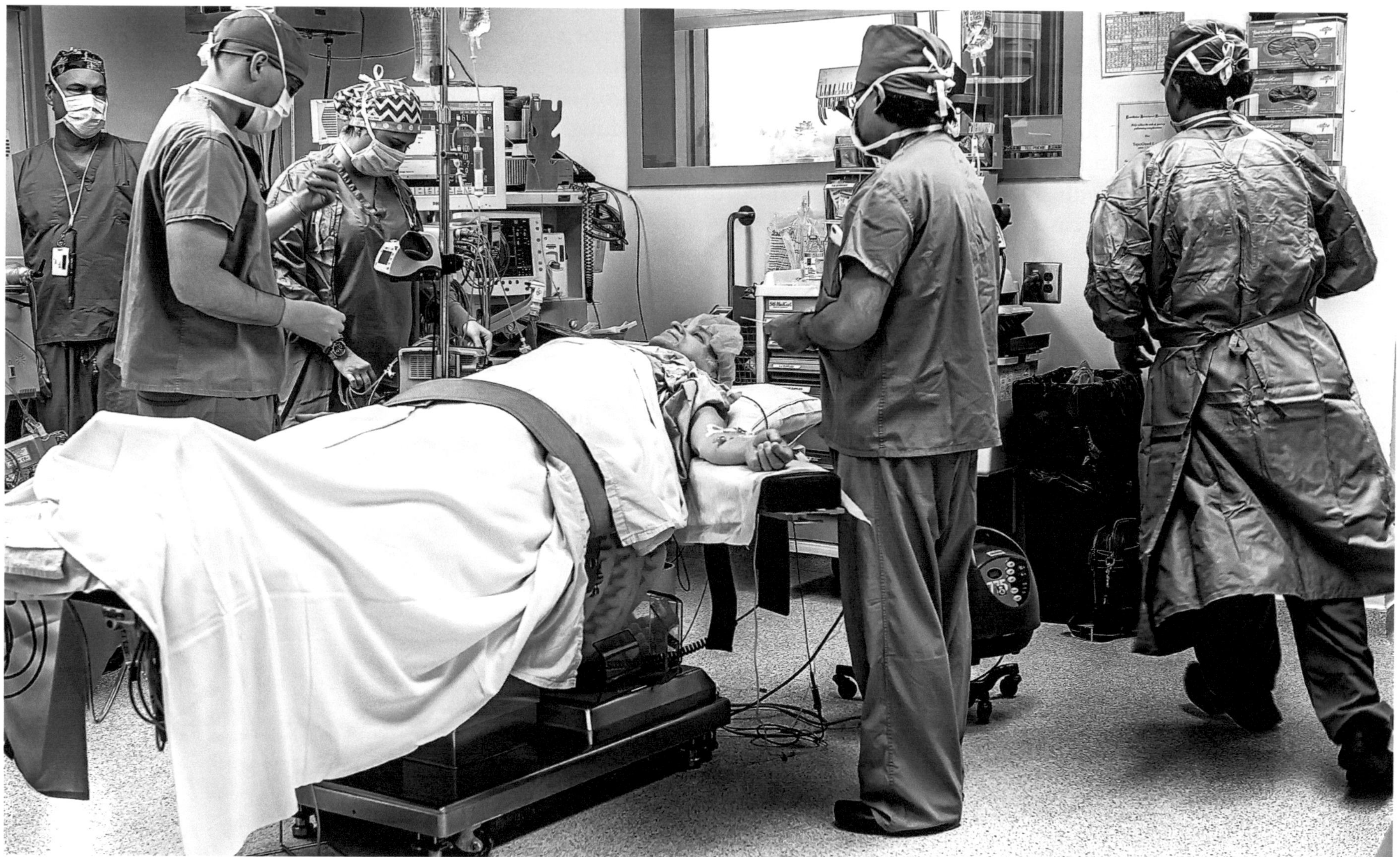

Patient identification checklist with cardiac surgeon

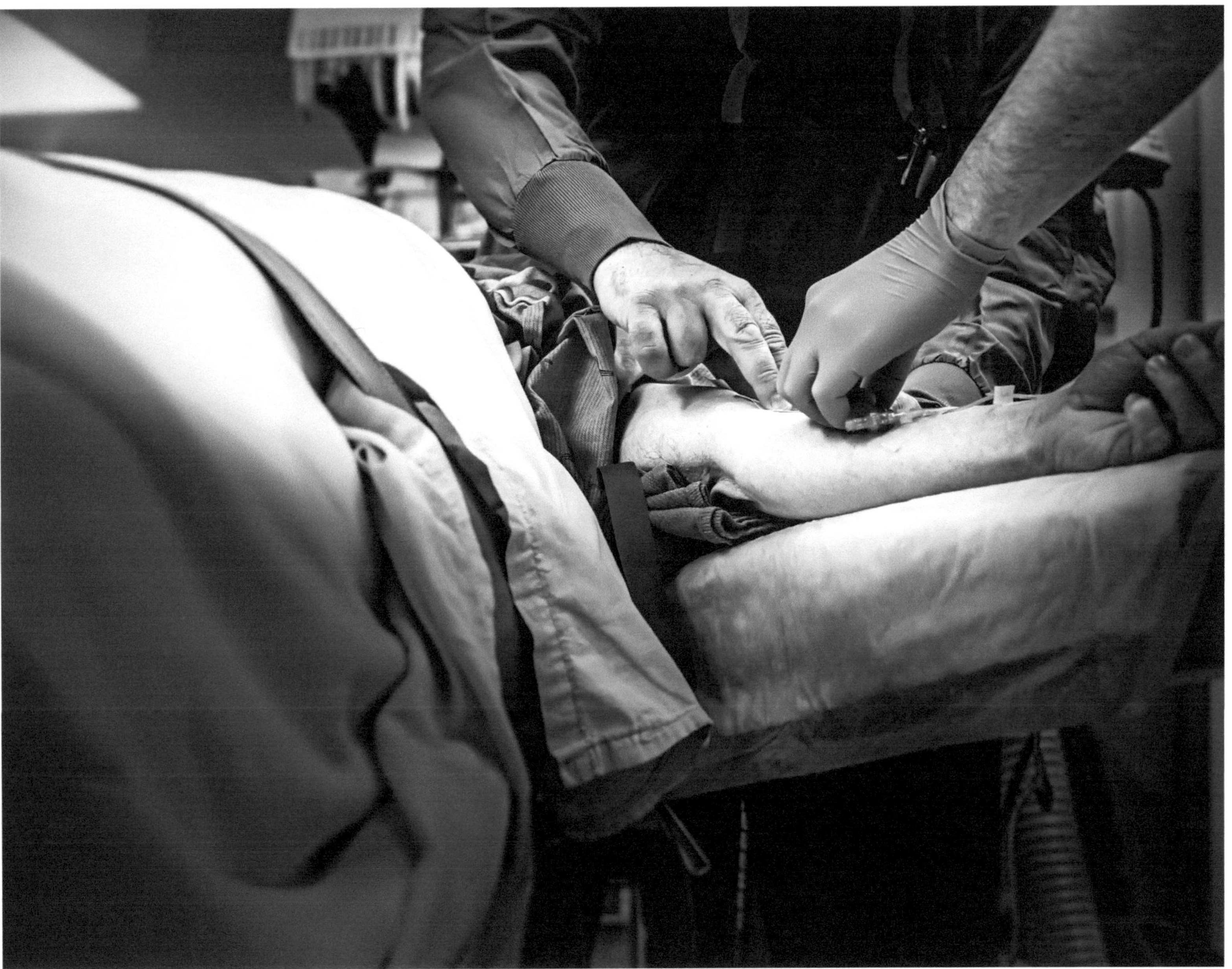

Intravenous line insertion

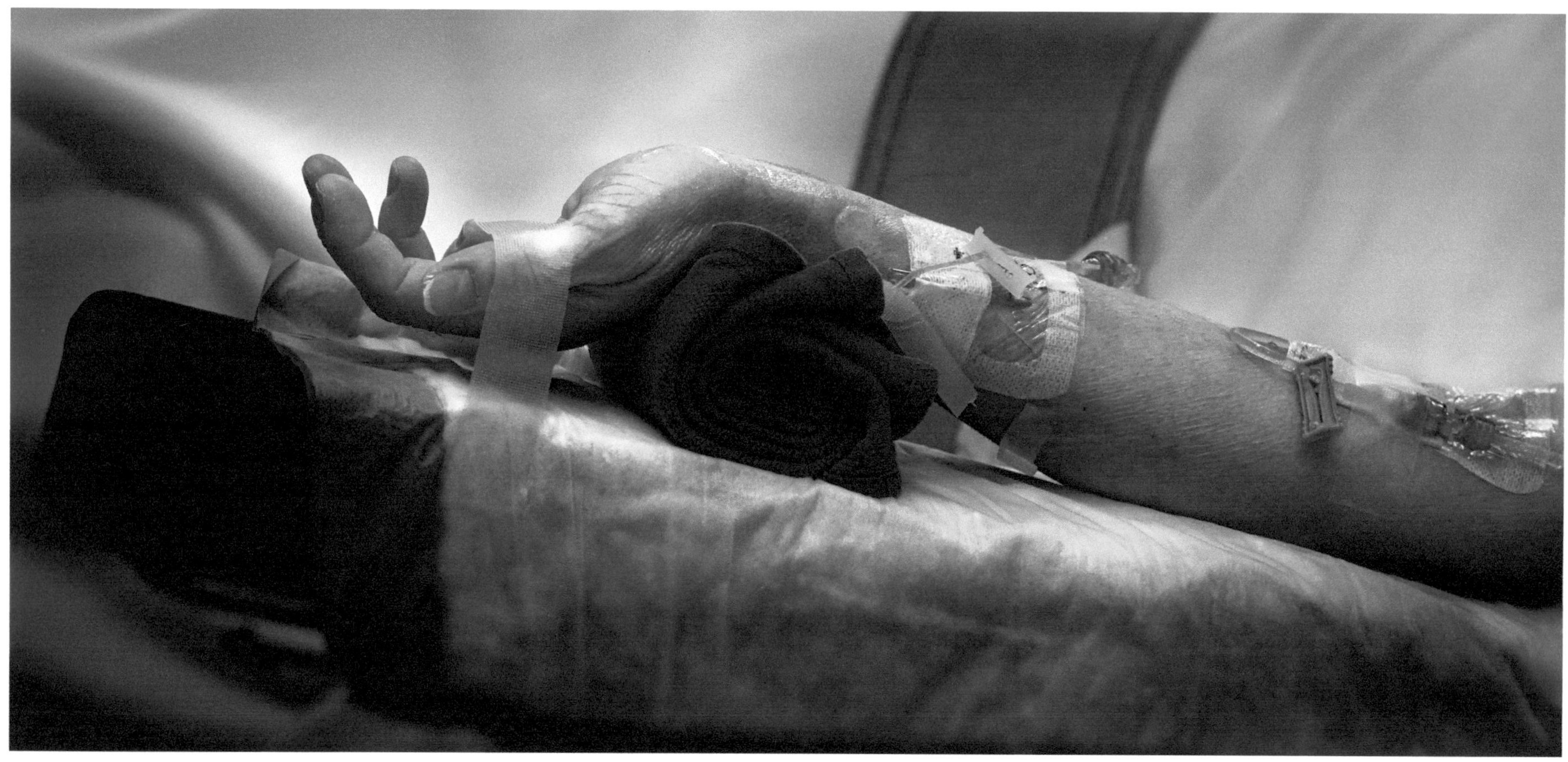

Intravenous lines inserted, and wrist is prepped for arterial line

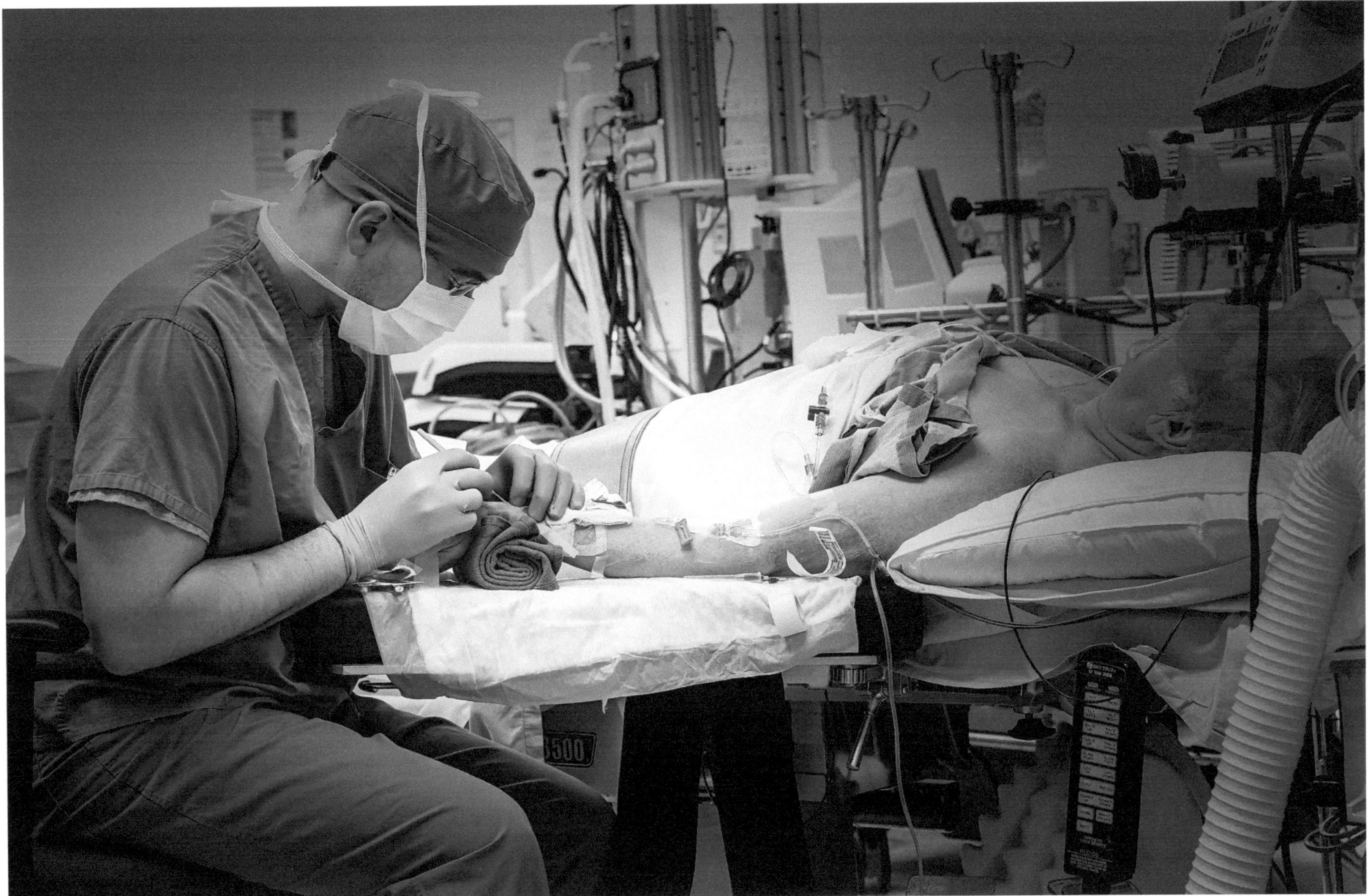

Radial artery discovery

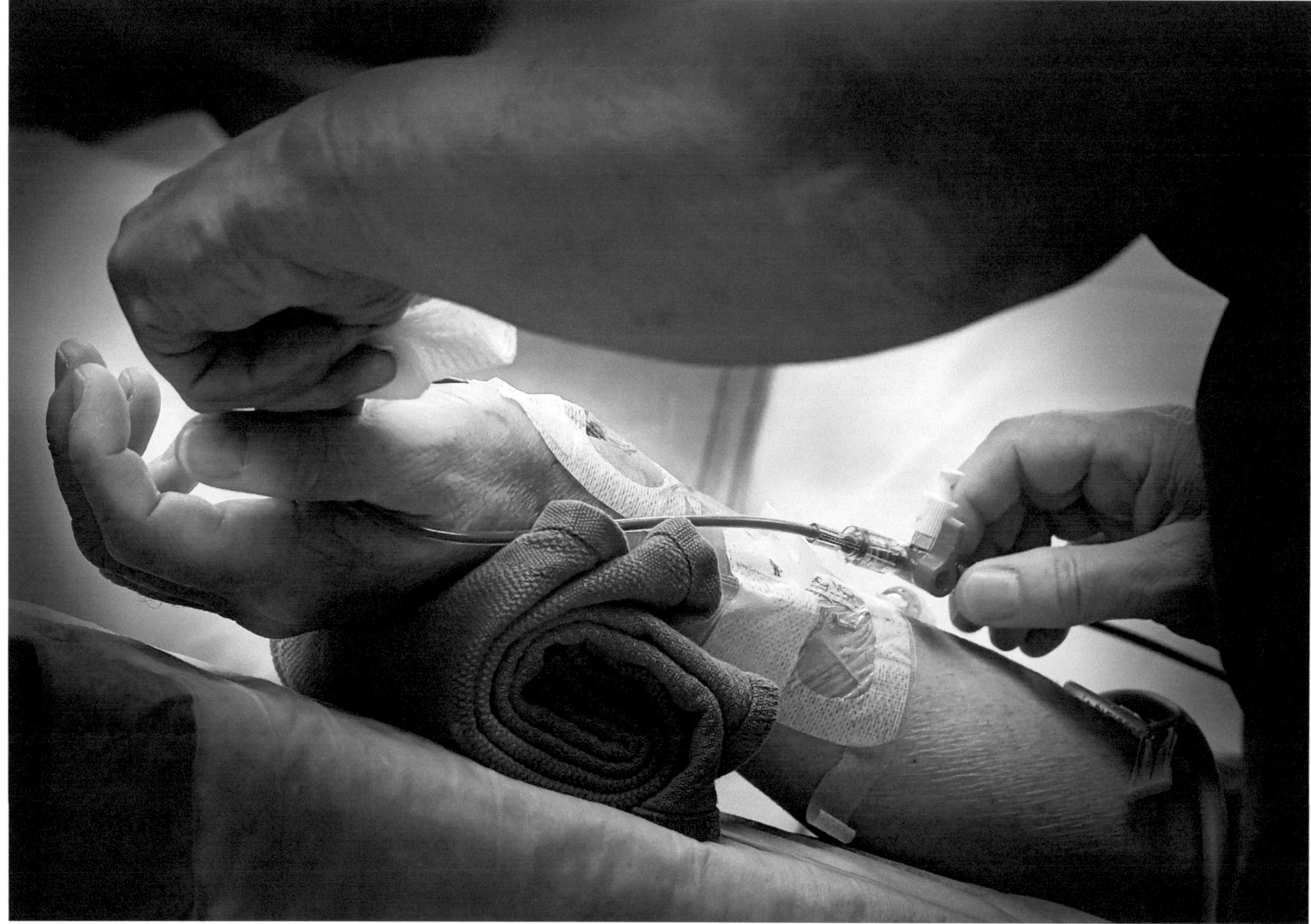

Radial artery is in place, marked by instant flow of bright red arterial blood in the arterial line

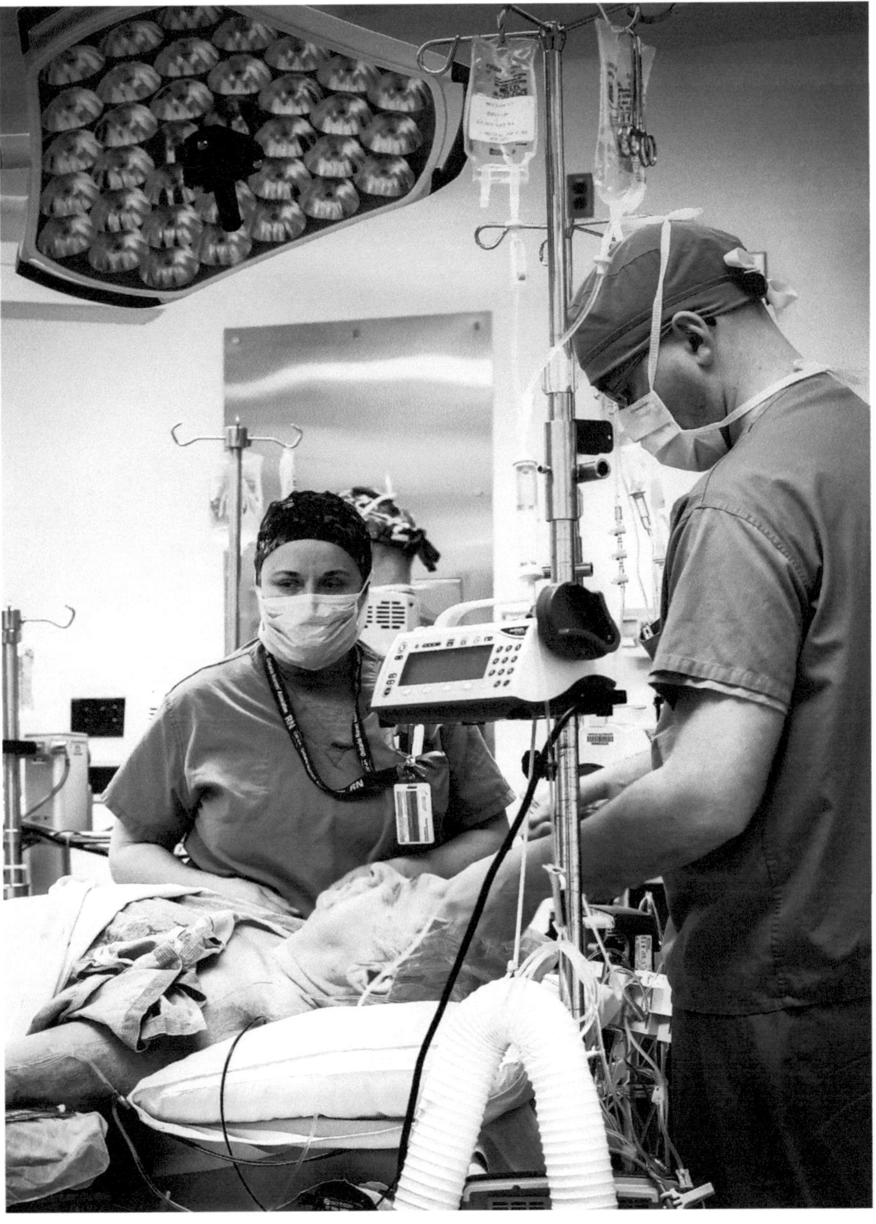

Sedation begins with anesthetist administering medications through the peripheral lines

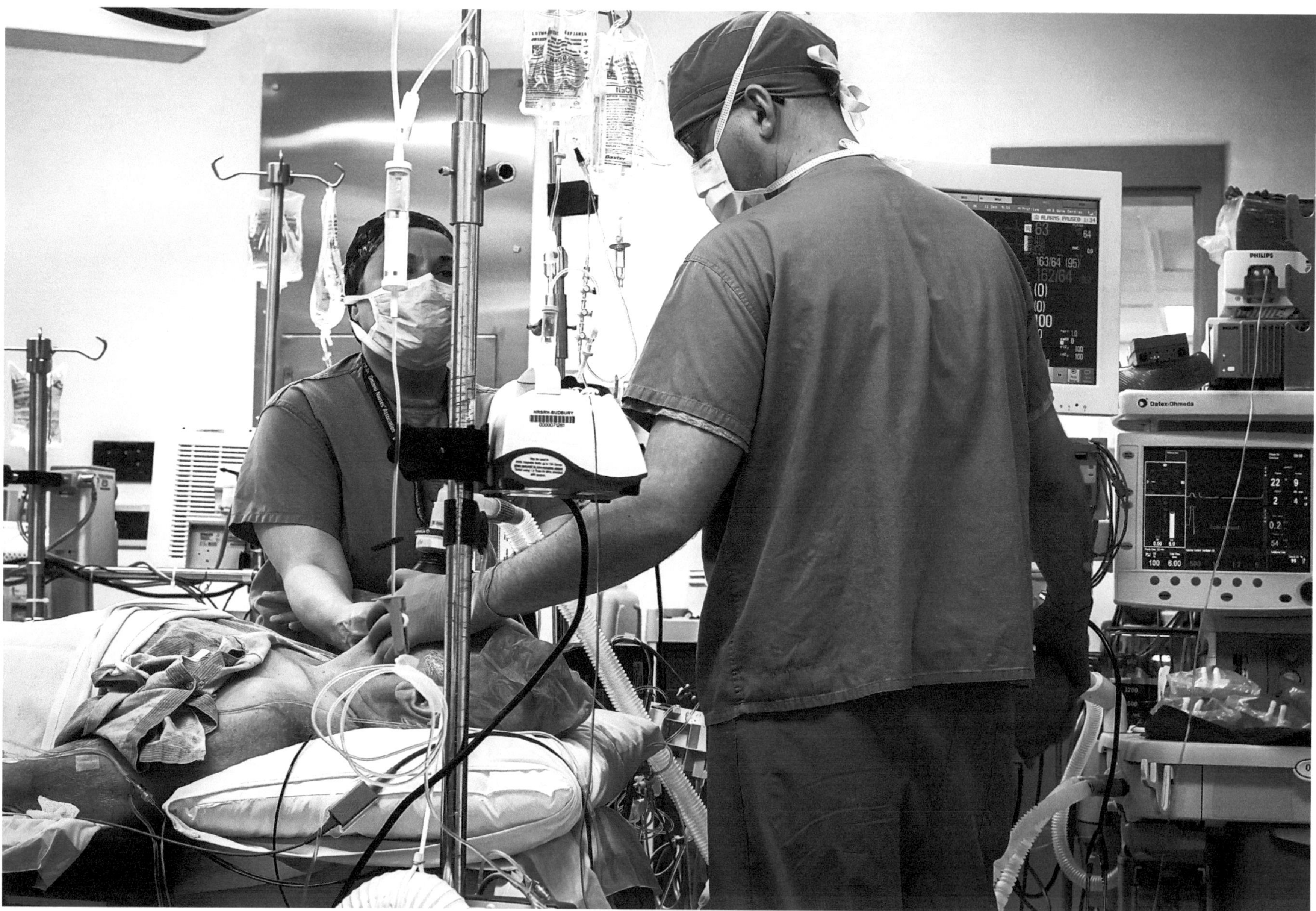

Administration of volatile gaseous anesthetic with the ventilation mask—patient drifting into deep sleep state

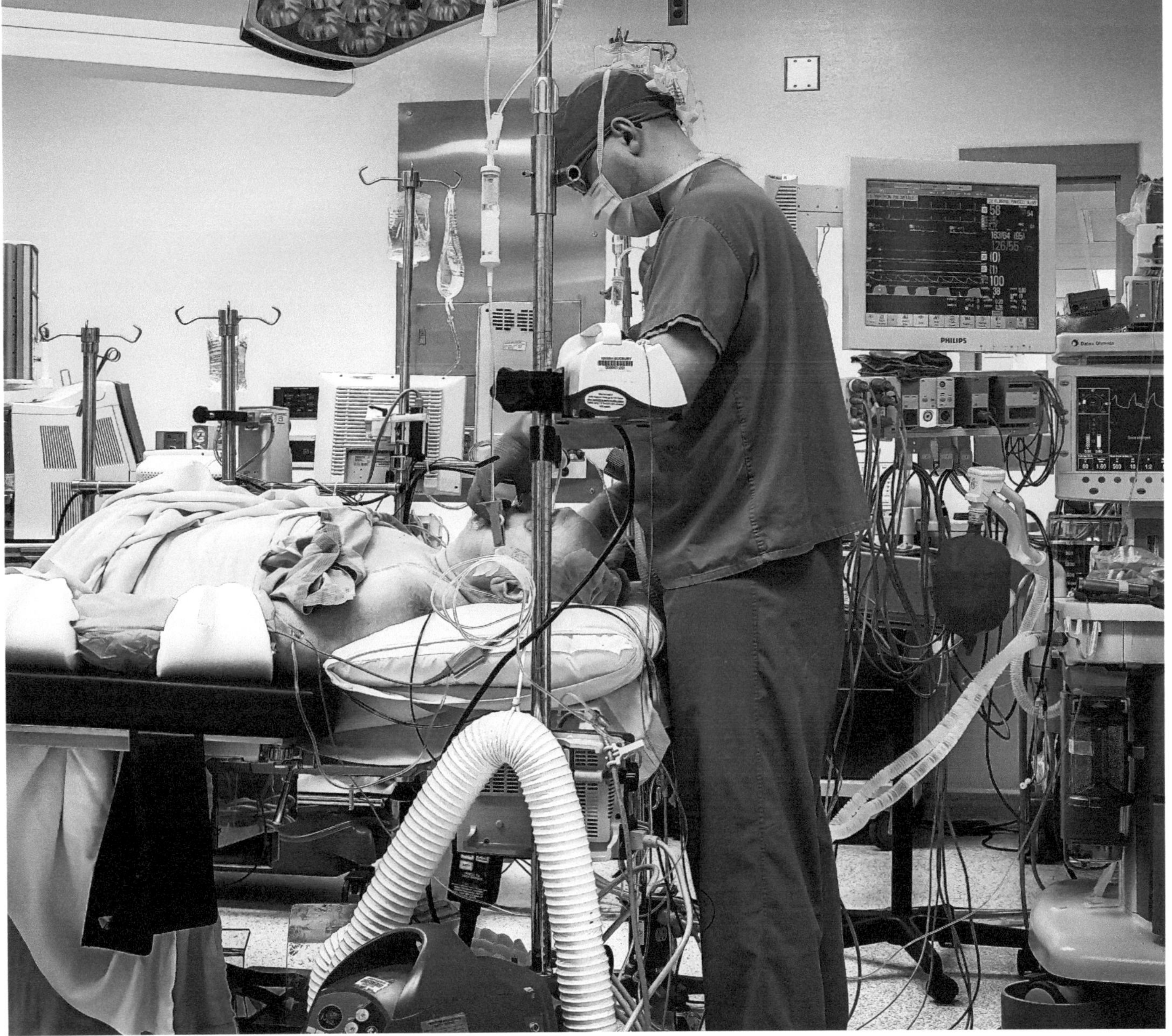

Anesthetist inserts a breathing tube connected to a ventilator, enabling external mechanical breathing

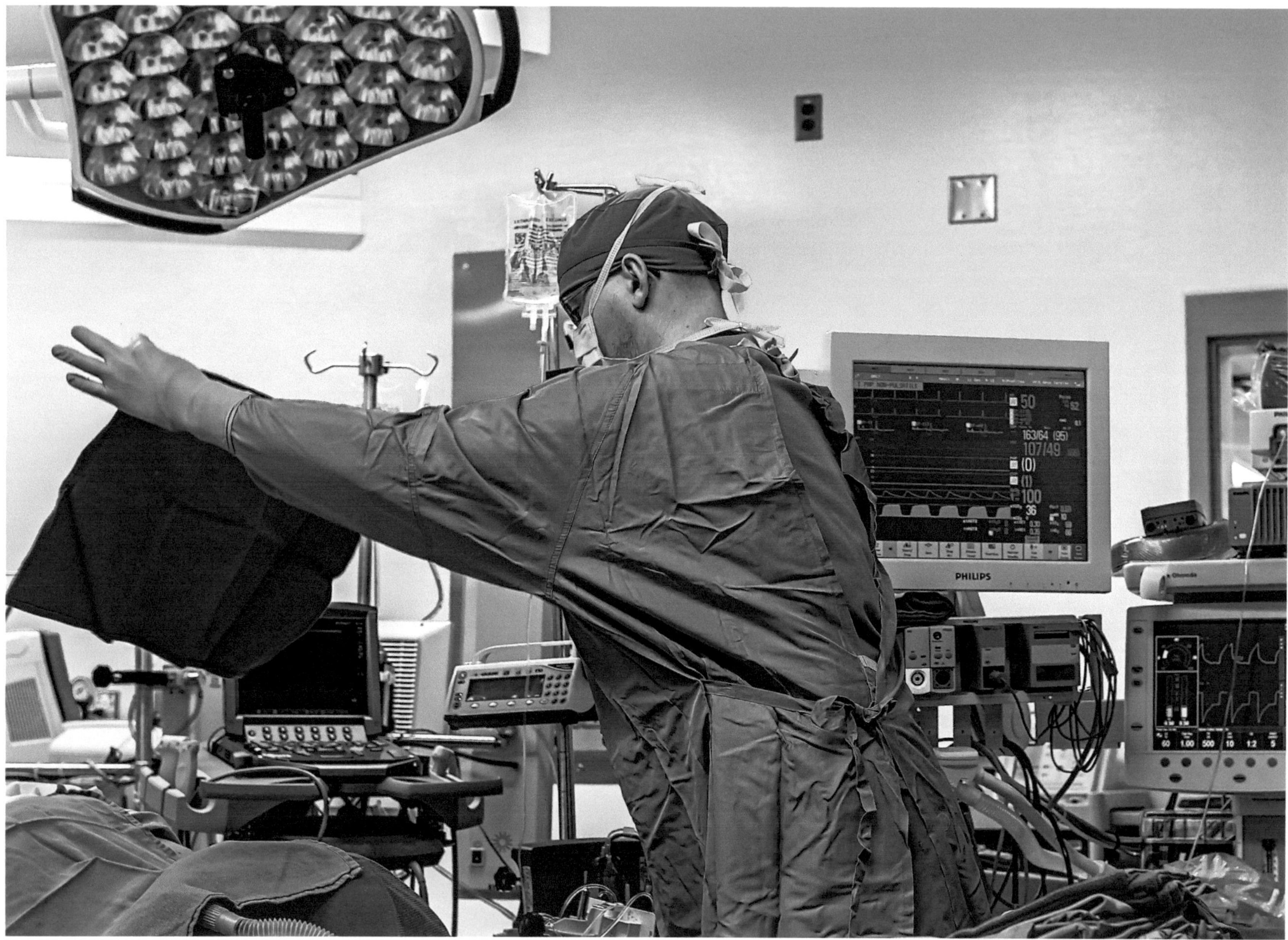

With breathing tube in place, patient is draped for the insertion of the central venous line through the jugular vein

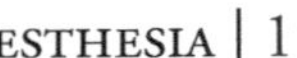

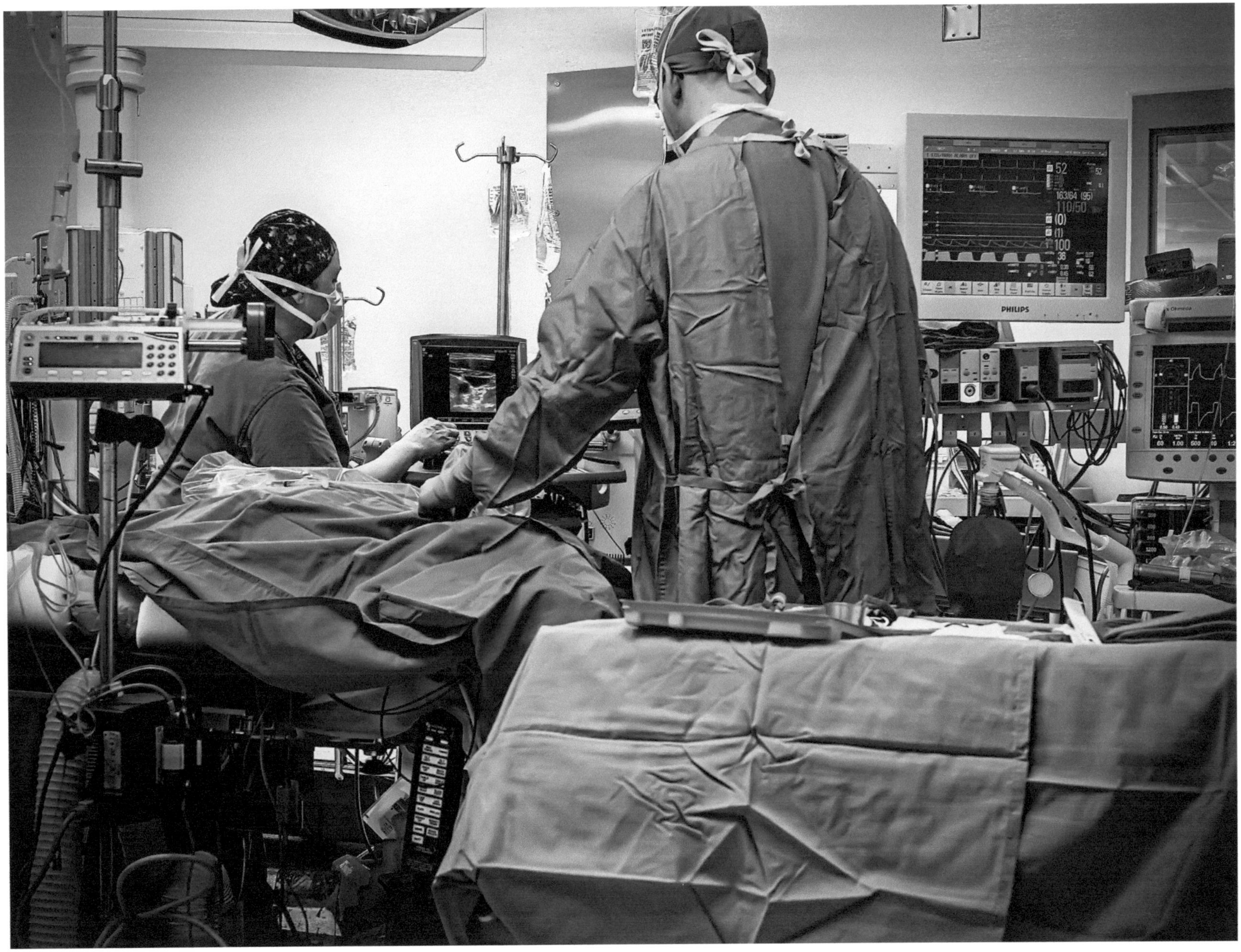

Ultrasound guided jugular vein discovery

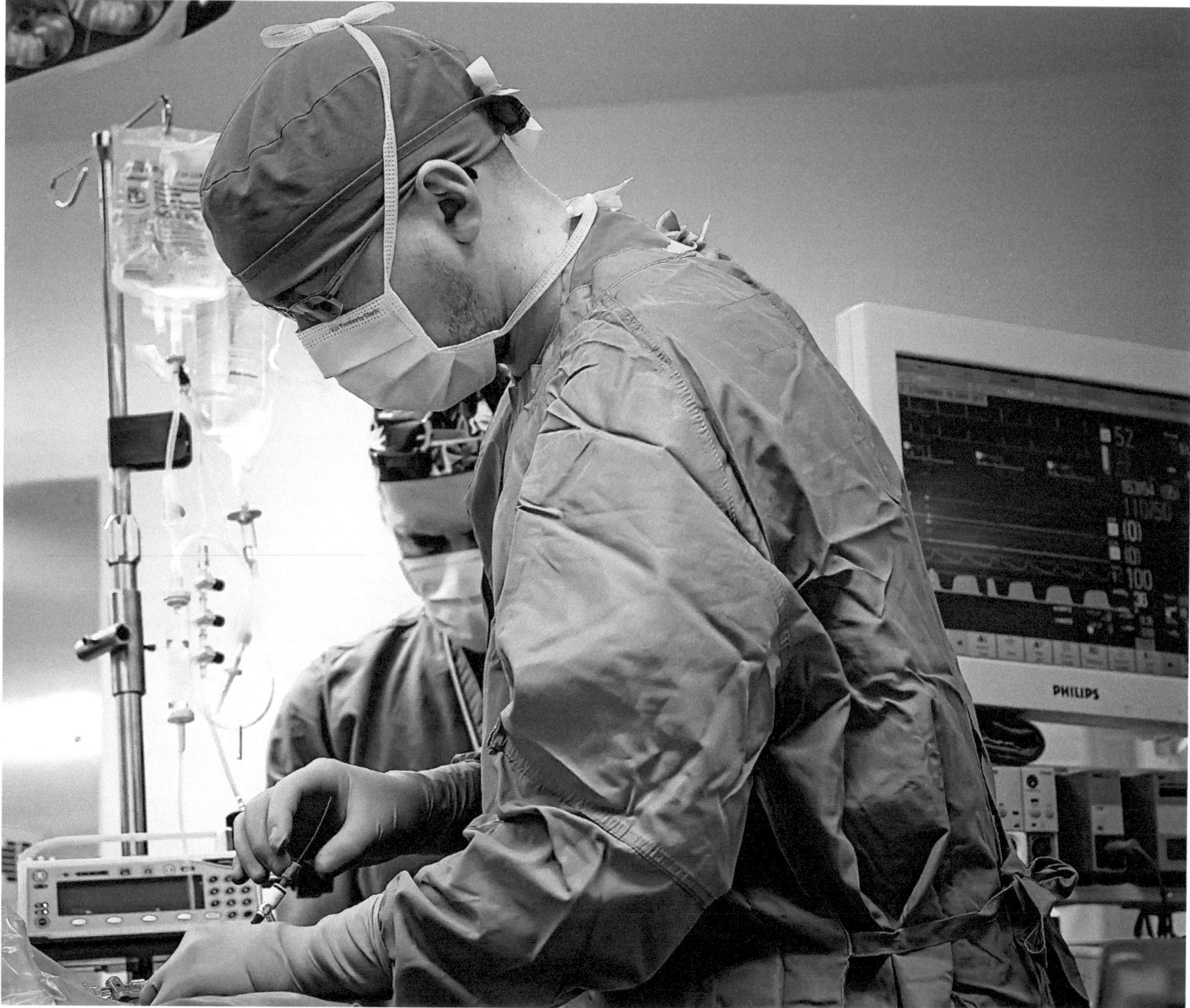

Central venous line going into jugular vein

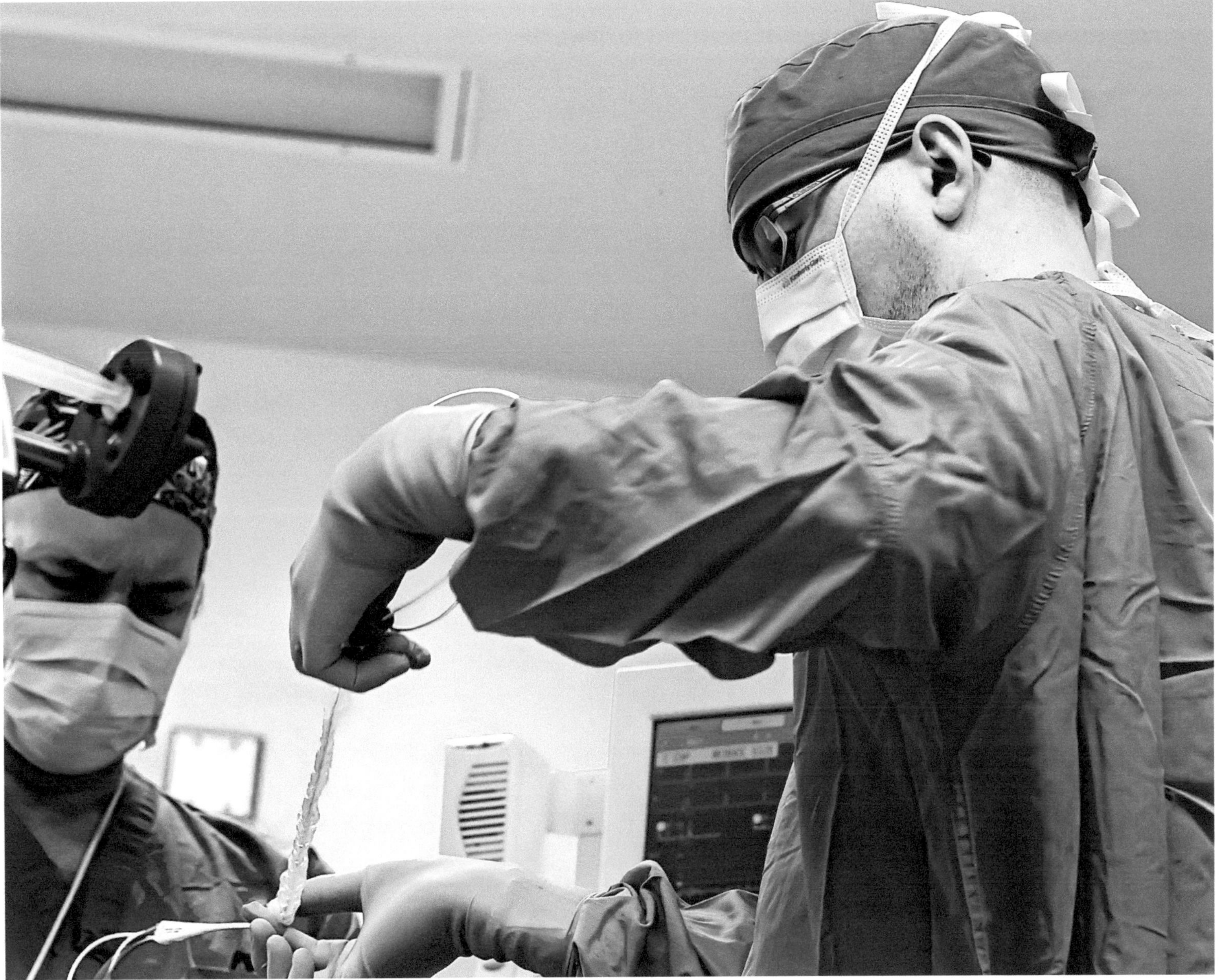

A Swan Ganz, a triple tube catheter system, used for voluminous influx of fluids and medications and for monitoring vascular pressures during the procedure, is inserted into the jugular vein

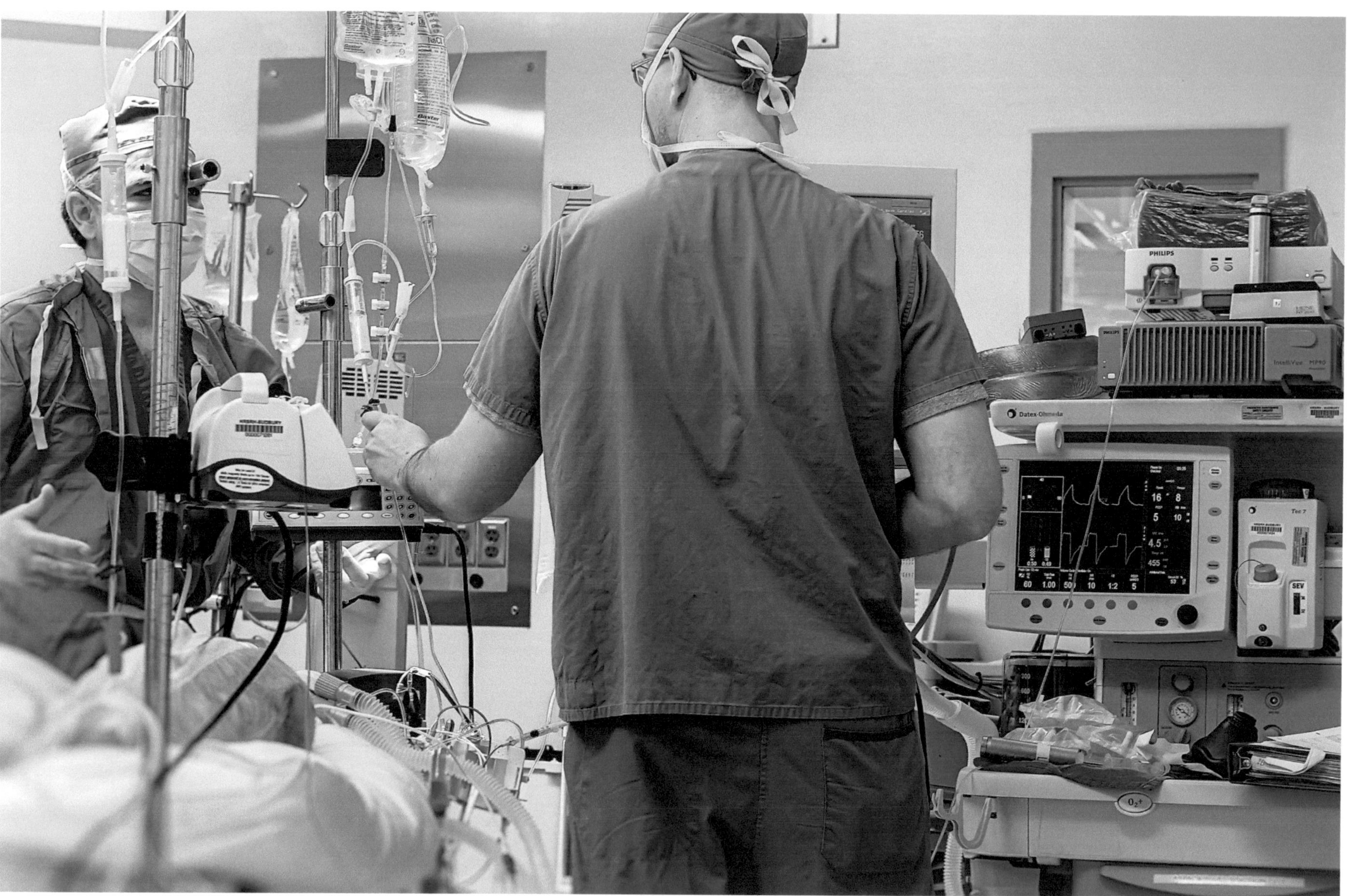

With central venous line, peripheral venous and arterial lines, and breathing tube in place, anesthetist drips medications and fluids into the venous lines; vascular pressures being monitored on screen

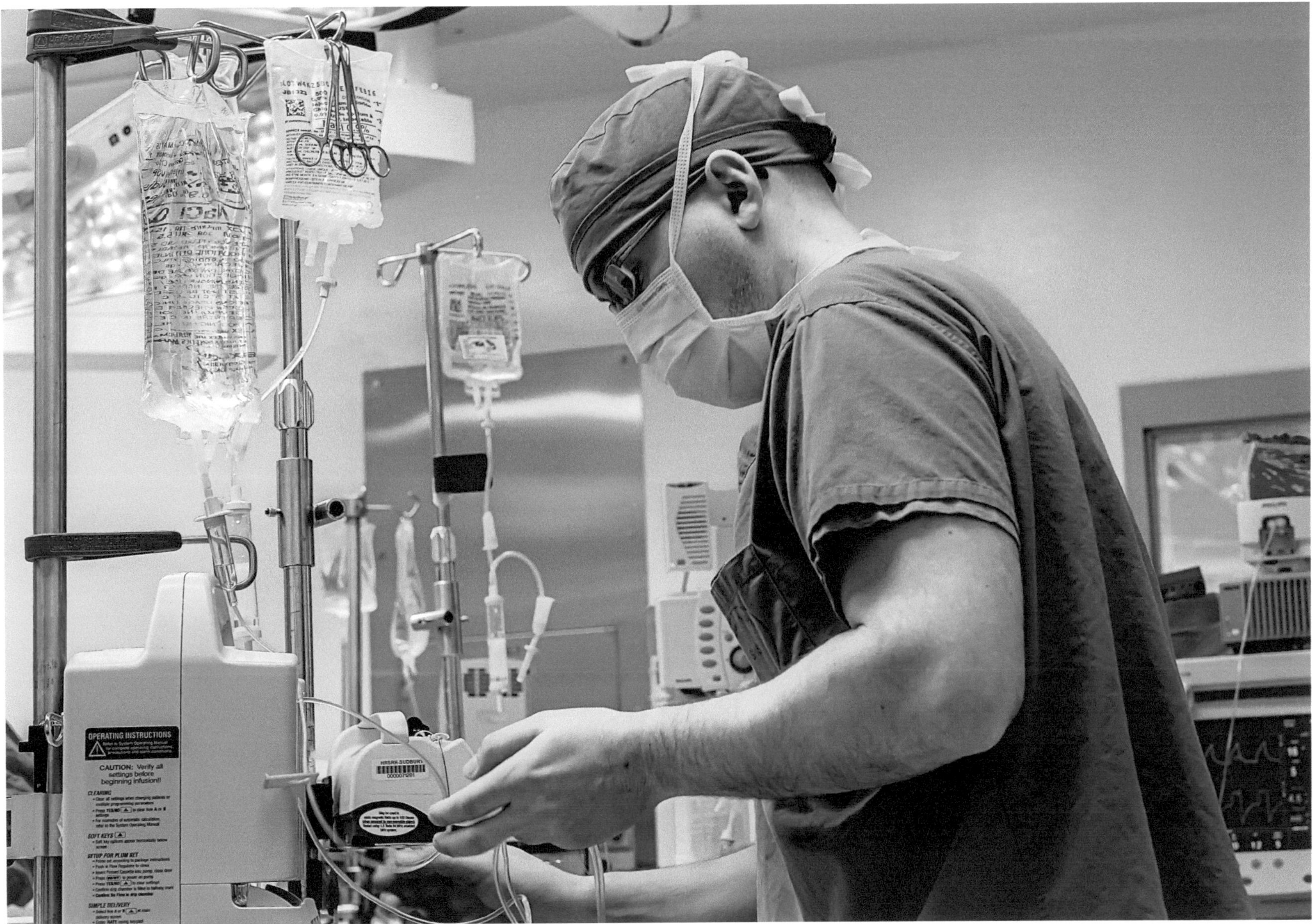

Fluids dispensed into venous lines through a machine monitoring fluid volumes

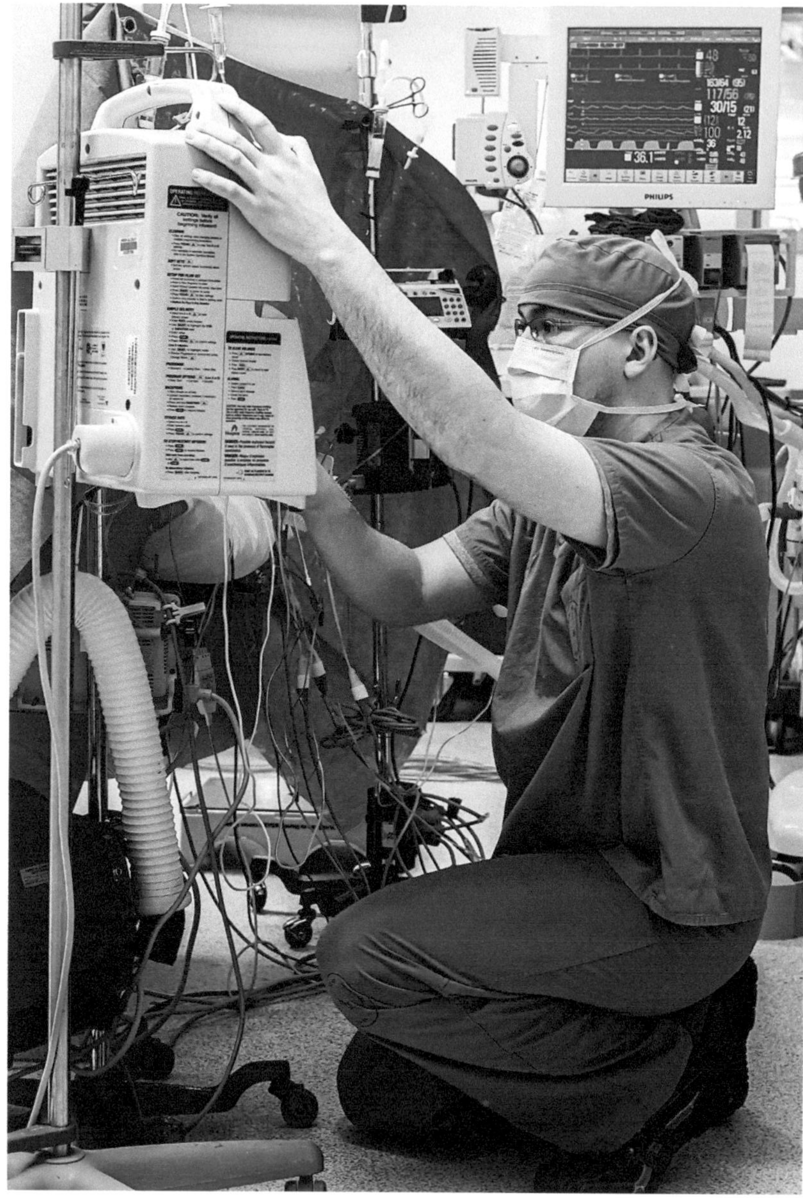

Anesthetist monitoring critical flow rates of fluids being infused

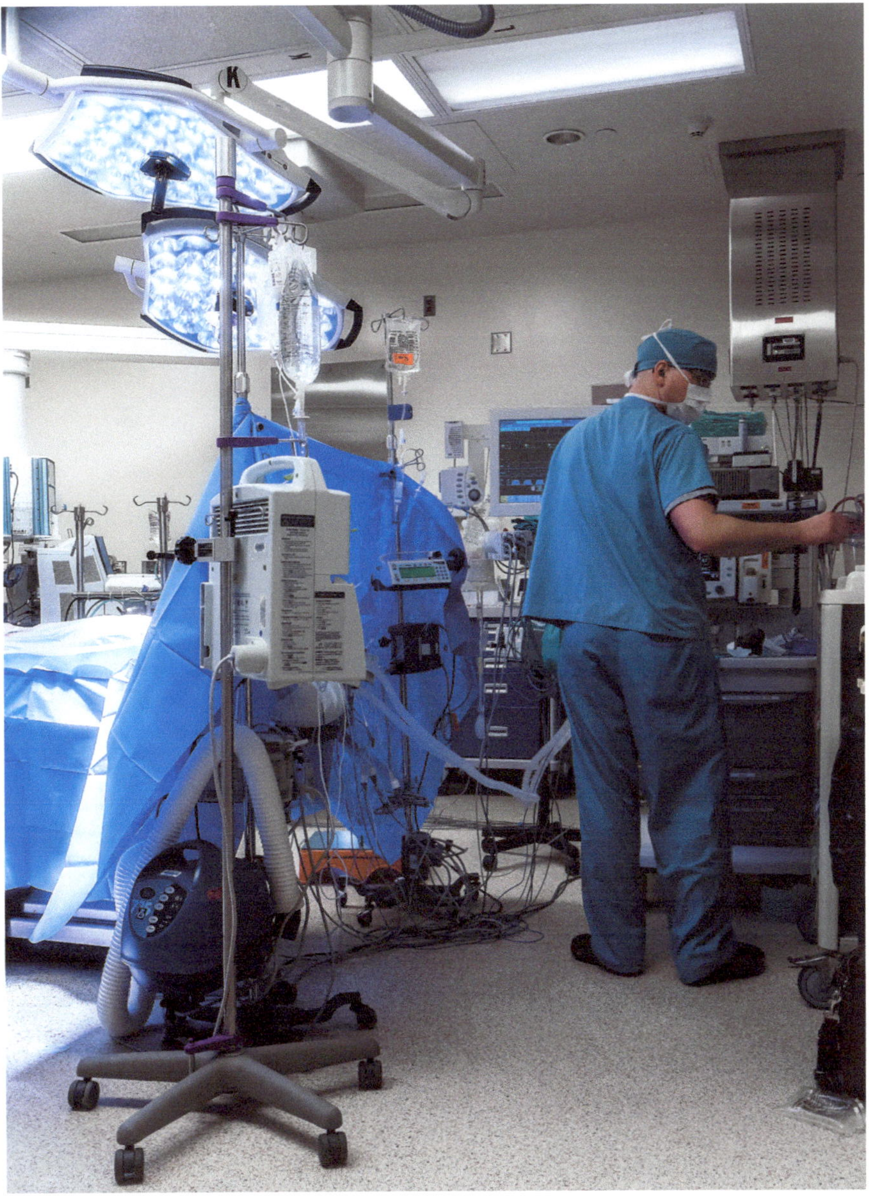

Patient in deep sleep state; patient's skin surface is sterilized with solution and drapes mounted; anesthetist monitoring patient's vital statistics

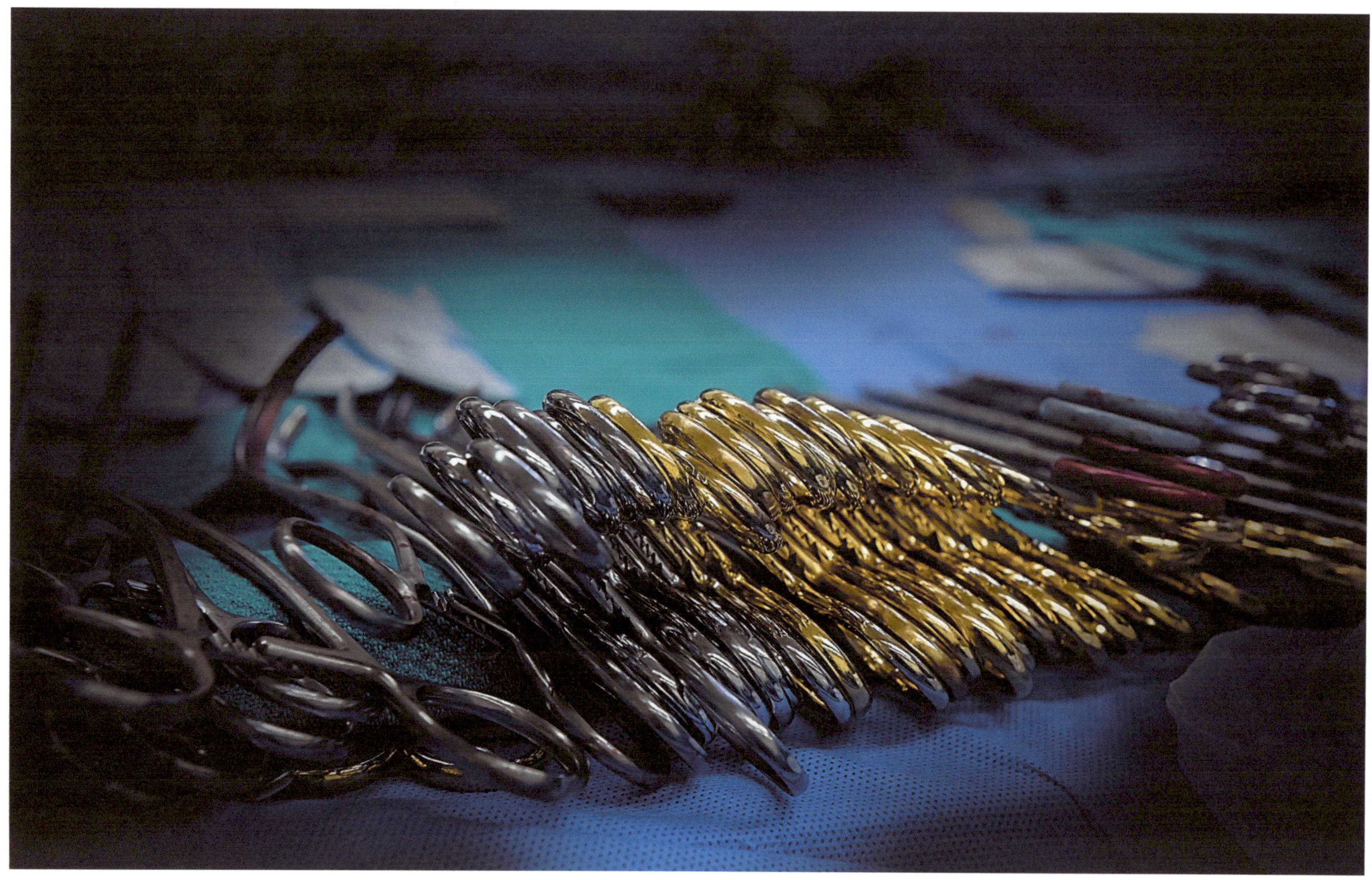

SURGERY BEGINS
Graft Harvesting

With patient asleep, enter the surgeons and surgical assistants, one by one into the operating room, with their forearms held up, out and extended. Each surgeon approaches the nurse, who holds in her hands the sterile operating gown with which she dresses the surgeon—first through the sleeves on the extended arms, he hands her the tie, twirls to wrap the gown around him and ties the tie in front. As I sat in the far corner of the operating room in oblivion, I was quite struck by this rhythmic routine. In my mind, they appeared akin to rock stars, one by one entering the operating room with nurses bustling around them before the show began. Concentration is immense, there is no talking, and each person knows what is next. Once clad in gowns, the nurse hands each one operating gloves. The surgeons take their positions around the patient on the table. Surgery begins.

At this stage, it is appropriate to understand the overall cardiac anatomy and function in order to follow the purpose and reasoning of various stages of the surgery. I will try to present the cardiac blood flow mechanics in simple terms. The heart is a powerful organ and maintains blood circulation throughout the body. It beats 100,000 beats a day or 2.5 billion times over a 70-year life span. An average male heart weighs around ten ounces, while a female heart is around eight ounces.

The heart, a mechanical pump, consists of two pumps, the right pump and the left pump. Each pump consists of two chambers, the atrium and the ventricle. The atrium is the filling chamber, while the ventricle is the pumping chamber. The right pump consists of the right atrium and right ventricle, and similarly, the left pump is made up of the left atrium and the left ventricle. Each pump has discreet functions. The function of the right pump is to pump impure, or de-oxygenated blood through to the lungs, while the function of the left pump is to pump pure oxygenated blood for transport to the body tissues. Veins, in general, carry de-oxygenated (venous) blood toward the heart, while arteries carry oxygenated blood away from the heart to the tissues.

The patient's right pump collects impure venous blood in the right atrium through two large collector veins. The superior vena cava (SVC) from the upper body above the neck and the inferior vena cava (IVC) brings blood from the lower body. Both drain into the right atrium. Blood in the right atrium enters the right ventricle through the tricuspid valve. The heart ejects blood from the right ventricle through the pulmonary valve into the pulmonary artery, which carries the blood to the lungs for purification (Illustration 1).

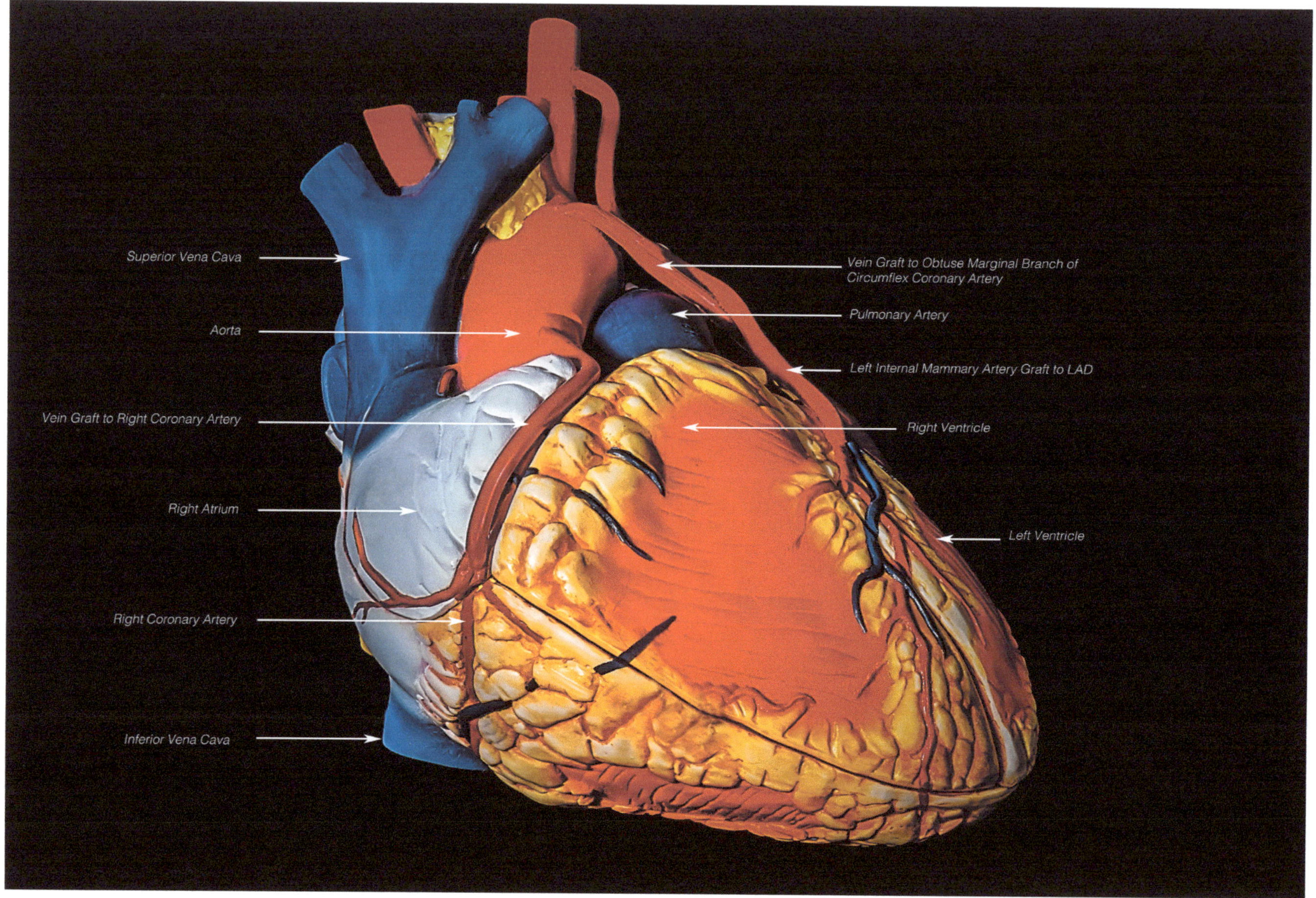

Illustration 1: View of the right side of the heart, showing the right pump. De-oxygenated blood from the body drains into the right atrium through the superior and inferior vena cava, into the right ventricle, and is ejected through the pulmonary artery to the lungs for oxygenation

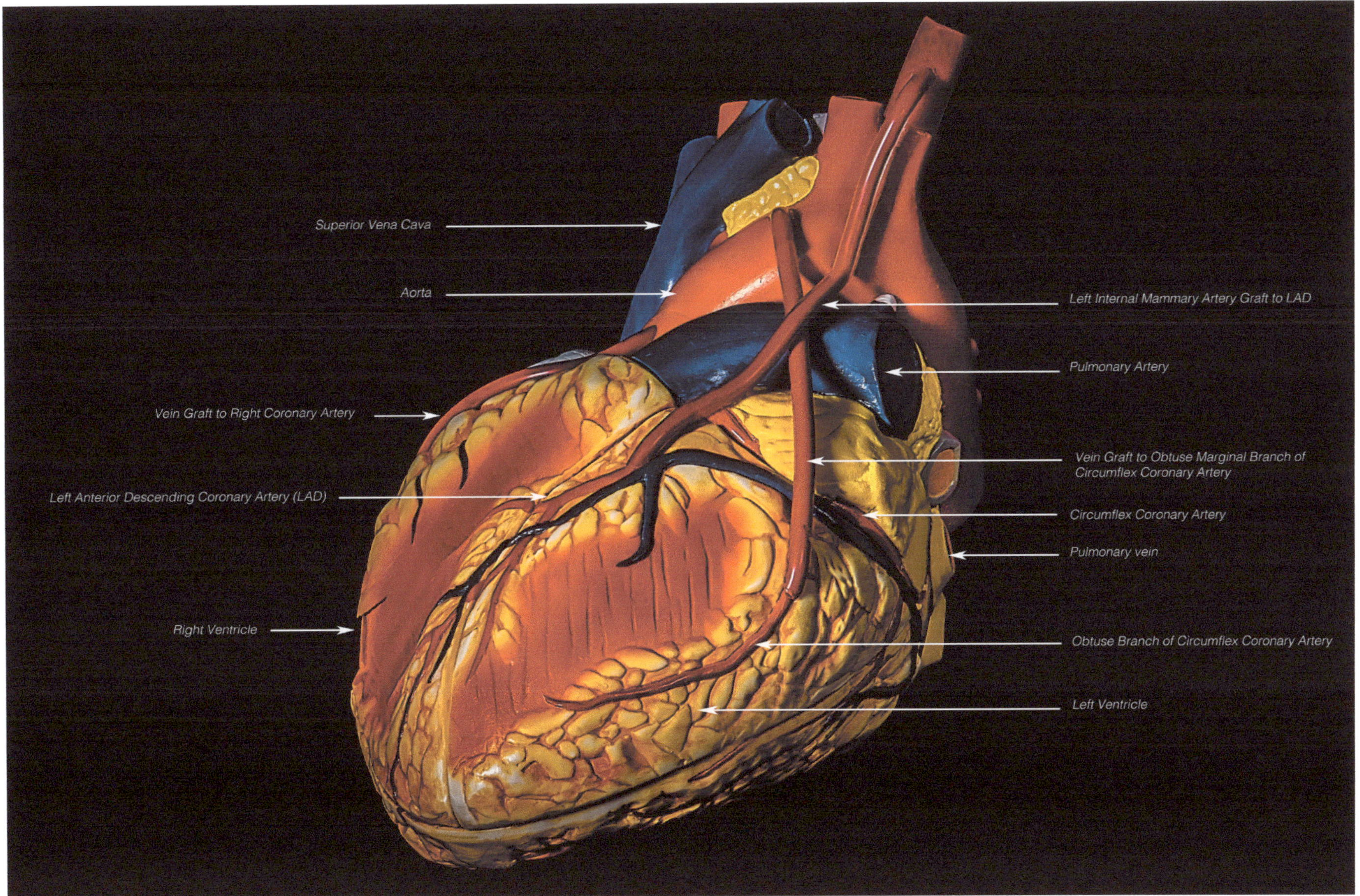

Illustration 2: View of the left side of the heart, showing the left pump. Oxygenated blood from the lungs drains into the left atrium through the pulmonary veins, into the left ventricle, and is ejected through the aorta supplying the body with fresh blood

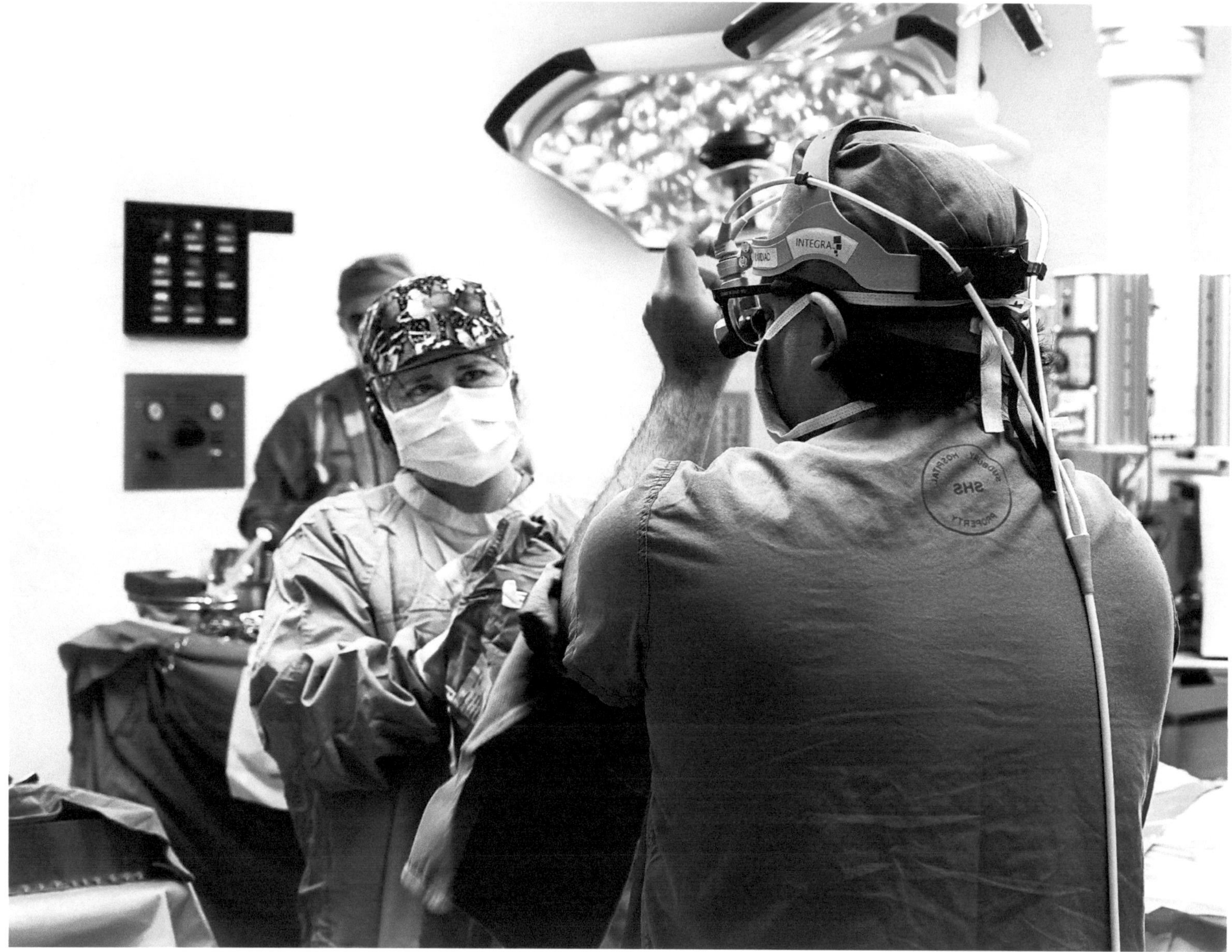

Dr. Garg being gowned for surgery

Lungs are the oxygenation center of the body, where oxygen exchange in the blood occurs. Oxygenated blood then drains into the left atrium through the pulmonary veins and then through the mitral valve into the left ventricle. From here, the heart pumps oxygenated blood from the left ventricle through the aortic valve to the aorta for circulation to the body (Illustration 2).

The lub-dub sound of the heart beat is the synchronous sound of the valves opening and closing in sequence, allowing fixed blood volumes (like packets of blood) to enter and exit the chambers in the heart. The mechanical pumping of the heart generates the blood pressure throughout the circulation system of the body. Systolic pressure refers to the blood pressure when the heart is pumping (contracting and ejecting blood), and diastolic pressure is when the heart is relaxing (dilating and filling). Pressures created in the heart are enormous, enough to squirt blood almost thirty feet.

The circulatory system transports blood throughout the body. The coronary circulation system, supplies blood to the heart itself in order to maintain its own functionality. This occurs through the right coronary artery and the left main coronary artery. Constant blood flow through these arteries is crucial in maintaining function of the cardiac muscle so that it can easily contract and relax, causing the heart to beat. When any one of these arteries or their branches occlude, blood is unable to reach areas of the cardiac muscle wherever these occluded arteries reside. This causes the muscle to die, resulting in a heart attack.

Risk factors for coronary artery disease include diabetes, hypertension, smoking, elevated blood cholesterol, and family history. Plaque build-up in the arteries eventually blocks blood flow through the arteries, causing chest pain, also known as angina, leading to myocardial infarction or heart attack. This causes areas of cardiac muscle to die, thereby reducing the overall heart function and its ability to pump effectively. Typical symptoms of coronary disease are chest pain and shortness of breath.

One treatment option for severe coronary disease is through surgical revascularization, or coronary artery bypass grafting (CABG). In other words, the cardiac surgeon creates a bypass with viable grafts of vein or artery from other areas of the body, bypassing the blockage, creating a new pathway for blood flow to revascularize oxygen-deprived areas of the heart. This is the first stage of surgery: graft harvesting.

Blood-conduits to bypass blockages on the heart can be either veins or arteries and are commonly referred to as grafts. Vein grafts are typically harvested from legs at the ankles, calves, or thighs. Arterial grafts are typically harvested from the artery on the inner surface of the chest wall, which normally supplies oxygen to the chest muscle. When an arterial segment is harvested from the chest wall, the body is normally able to compensate from other arteries in the region. Similarly, for veins harvested from the leg, other veins in the area compensate for the reduced blood-flow return to the heart, however it is a slower recovery. Typically, patients can expect leg swelling for several months after surgery. This is because blood collects in the leg due to reduced drainage until the body adapts to the vein deficit.

Shown in Illustrations 1 and 2 are the grafts constructed by the surgeon. The vein grafts are constructed with a connection from the aorta to the coronary artery in a region downstream to the blockage, thereby creating a bypass. The arterial Left Internal Mammary Artery (LIMA) graft, which naturally arises from a central arterial system, only requires one connection downstream to the blockage on the coronary artery.

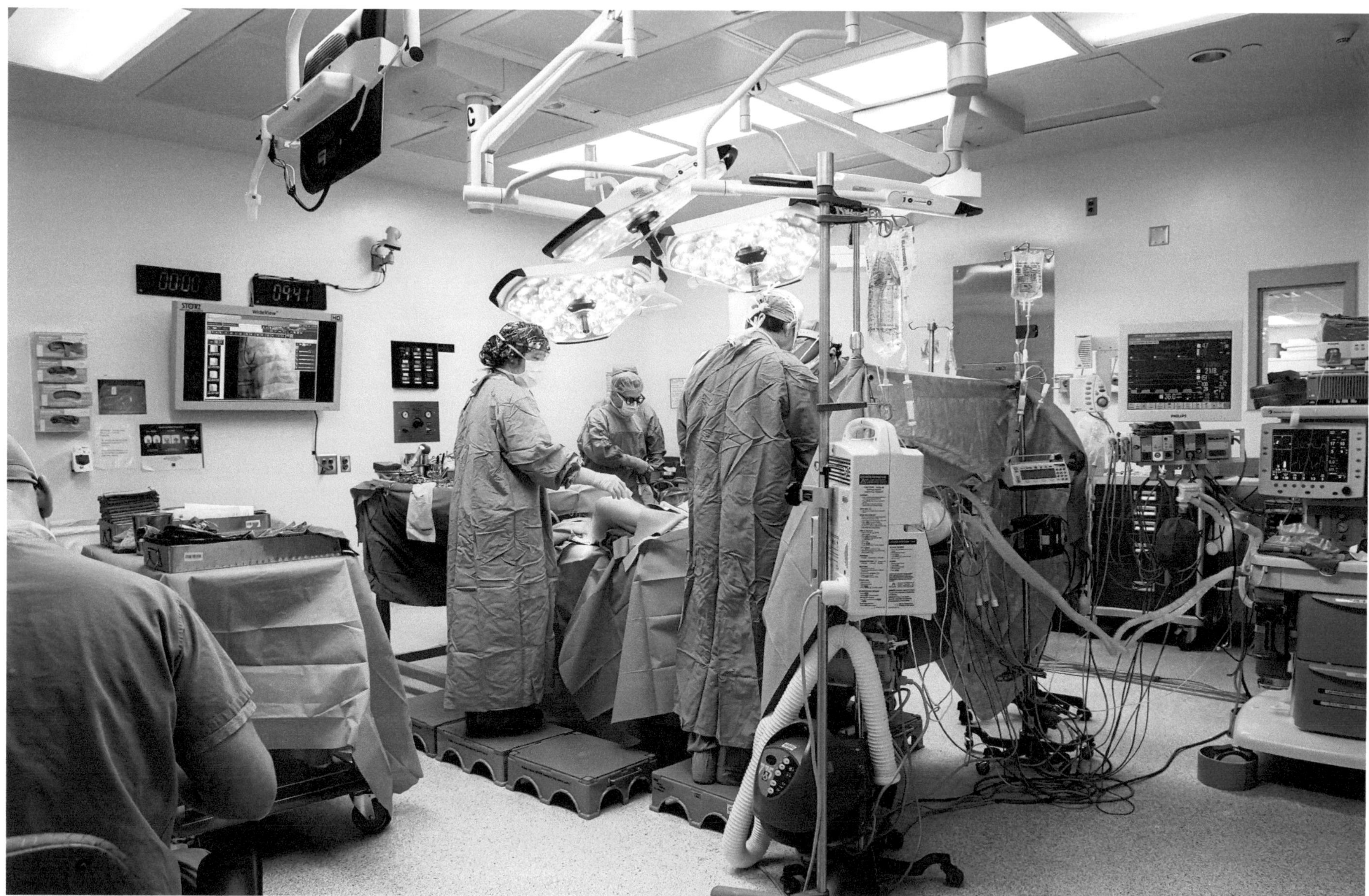

Doctors and nurses take their positions around the table

So why have arterial grafts in addition to vein grafts? Research has shown arterial grafts to have a longer patency rate of about 90% over a ten-year period, while vein grafts have a patency rate of about 60% over the same time period.[1] Longer viability of arterial grafts is likely due to an artery-to-artery connection, which is more natural than an artery-to-vein connection. It is for this reason the arterial graft is grafted to the most important vessel on the heart, the left anterior descending coronary artery.

In the photographs that follow, Dr. Garg and his surgical team begin with graft harvesting. His first assistant, cardiac surgeon Dr. Atoui, is seen harvesting the vein graft from the leg. Dr Garg, at the chest, begins by opening the chest and exposing the heart, followed by taking down the left internal mammary artery for the arterial graft. Assisting Dr. Garg is second assistant, Dr. Chow, who assists the lead surgeon at the chest. Also present is operating room nurse Chantal, who stands beside the instrument tray. Experienced in the operating room, she intuitively knows the instrument Dr. Garg calls for as he raises his hand. Each individual around the patient table is immersed in their role, all working in immaculate unison.

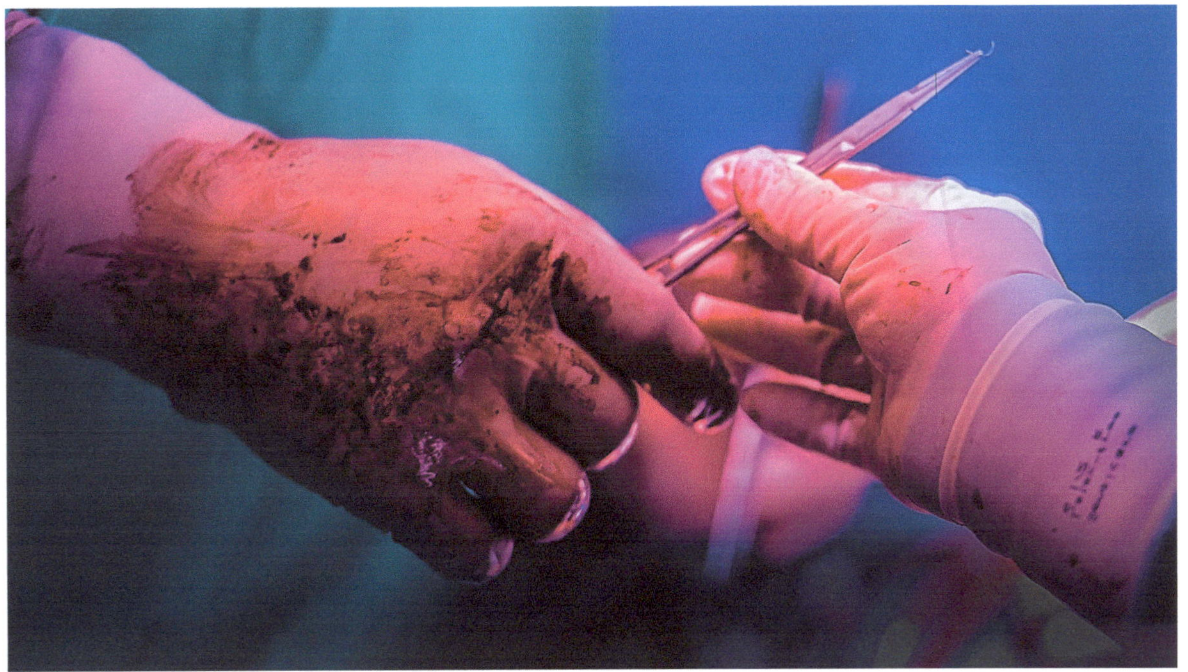

1 Goldman, Steven, et al. "Long-Term Patency of Saphenous Vein and Left Internal Mammary Artery Grafts after Coronary Artery Bypass Surgery." Journal of the American College of Cardiology, vol. 44, no. 11, 2004, pp. 2149–2156., doi:10.1016/j.jacc.2004.08.064.

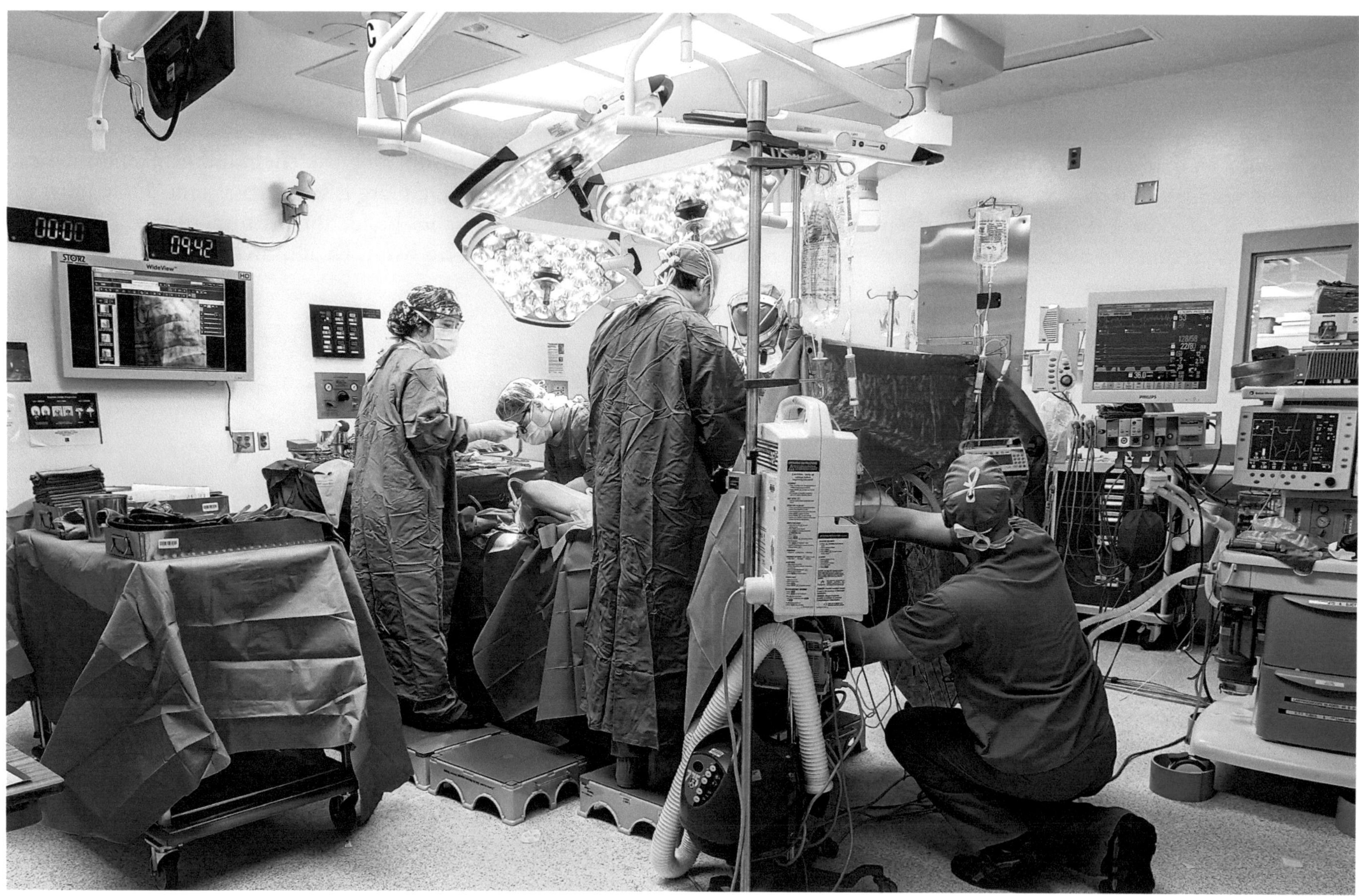

At the patient's head, on the right side of the chest, is lead cardiac surgeon, Dr. Garg, and on the patient's right leg is cardiac surgeon Dr. Atoui, first assistant. At the head on the left side of the chest is Dr. Chow, second assistant, and at the foot is operating room nurse Chantal, beside the instrument table. Dr. Stewart, anesthetist, monitoring patient vitals behind the operating table.

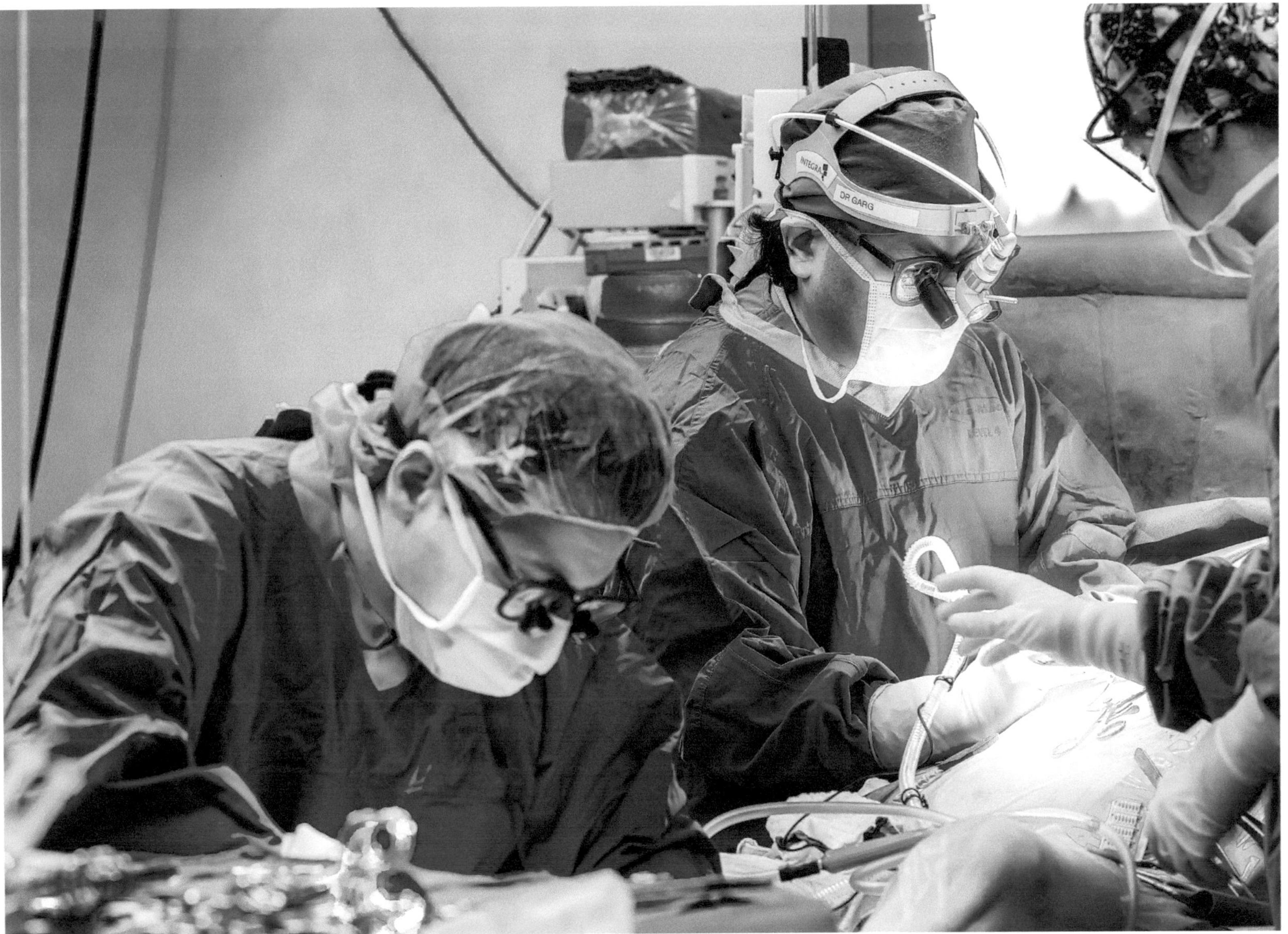

Dr. Garg, making a midline skin incision on the chest. The sternum is then opened and the heart is exposed. Dr. Atoui, at the foot, dissects the leg to harvest vein grafts.

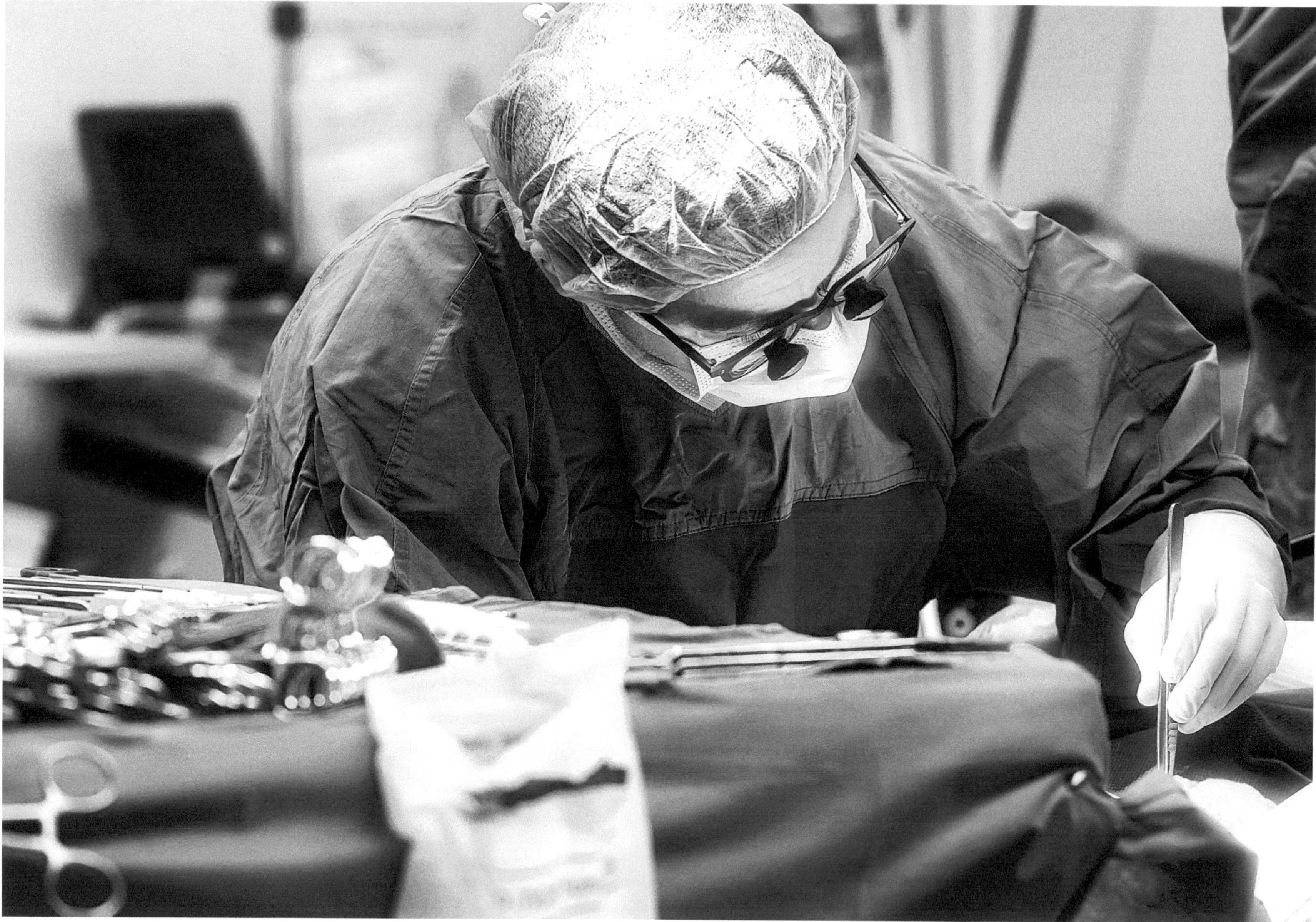

Dr. Atoui, dissecting the leg

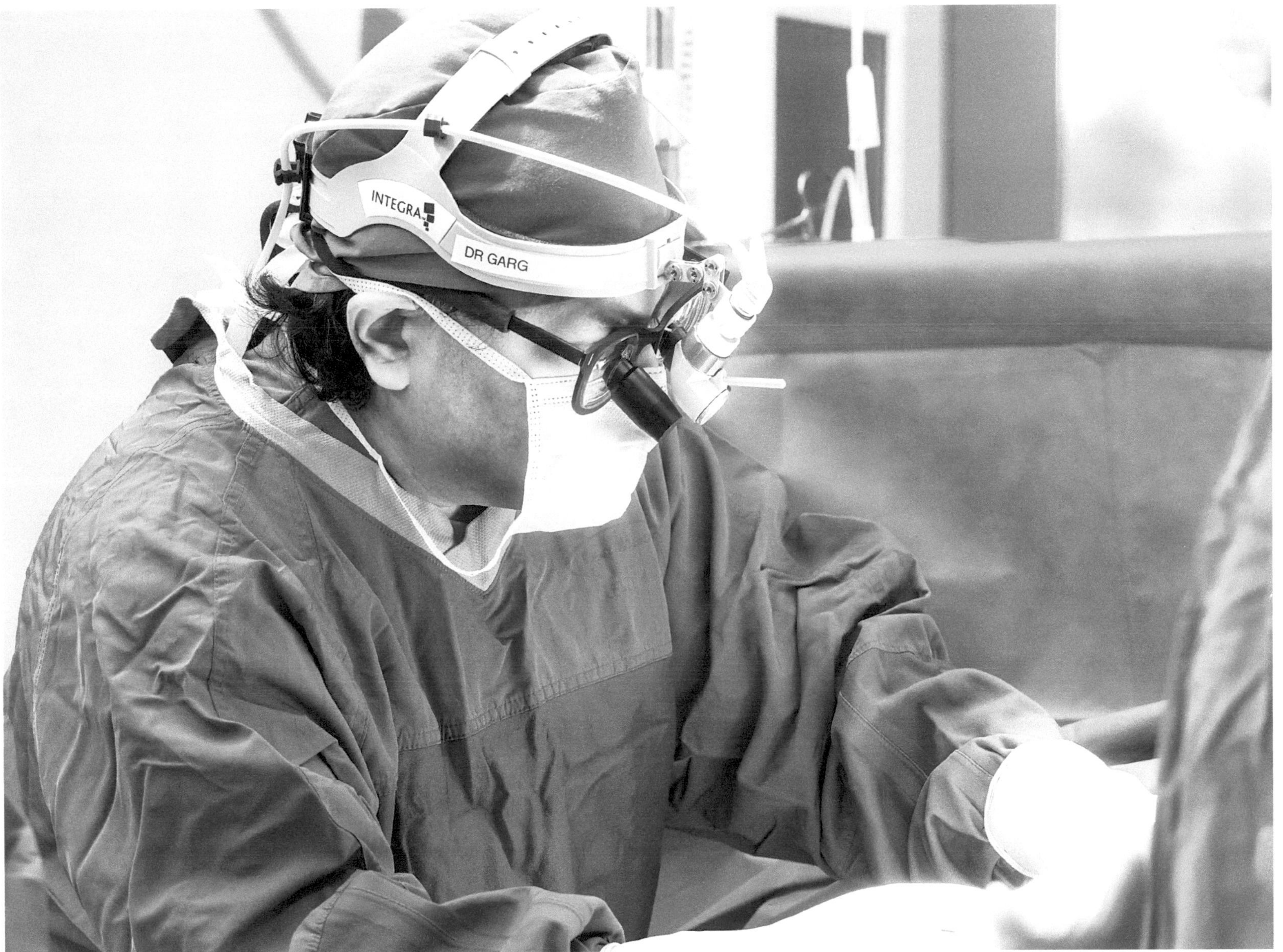

Dr. Garg, making the sternal incision

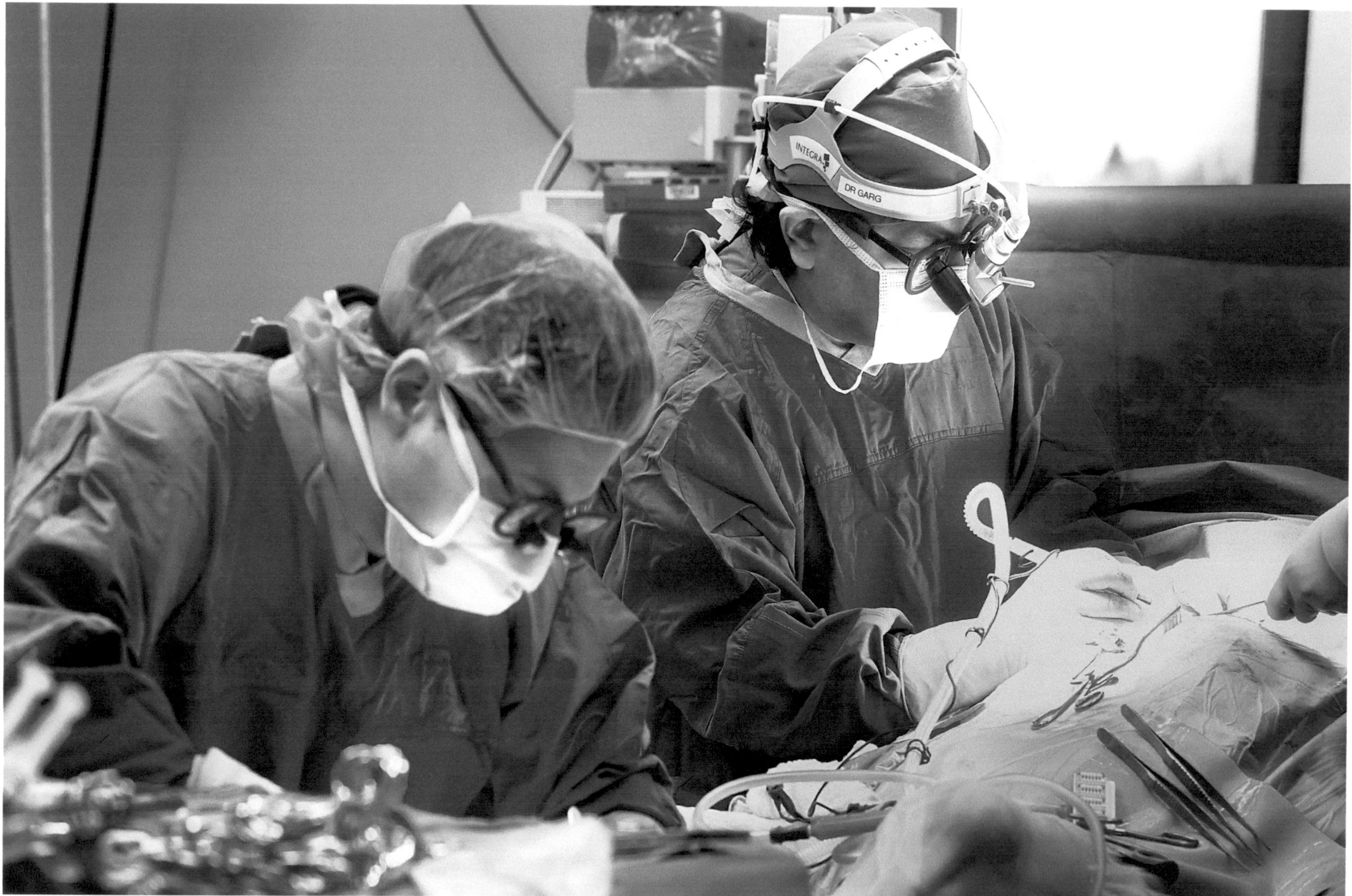

Dr. Garg, opening the chest, and Dr. Atoui, harvesting the vein

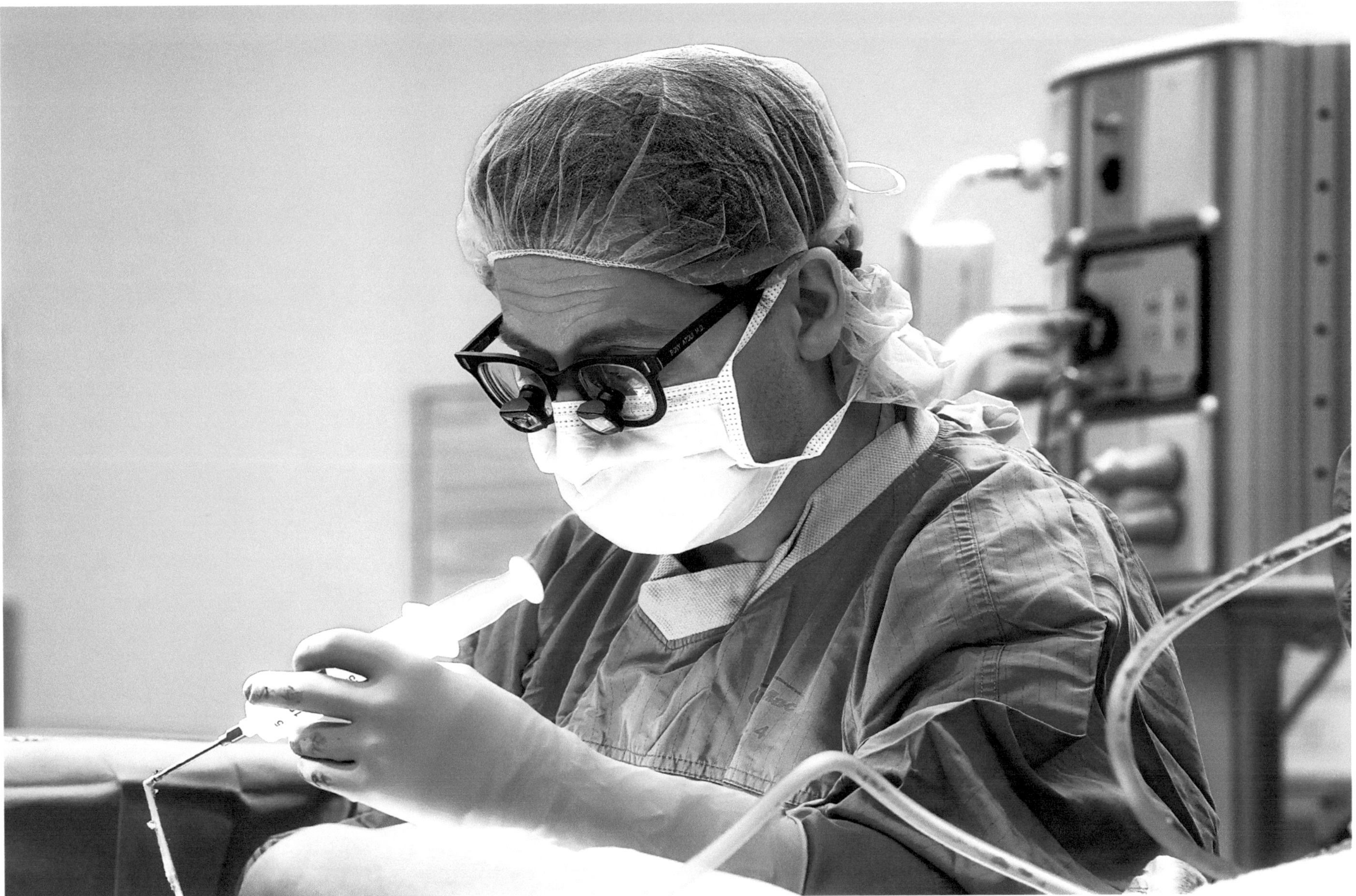

Dr. Atoui checking integrity of the harvested vein

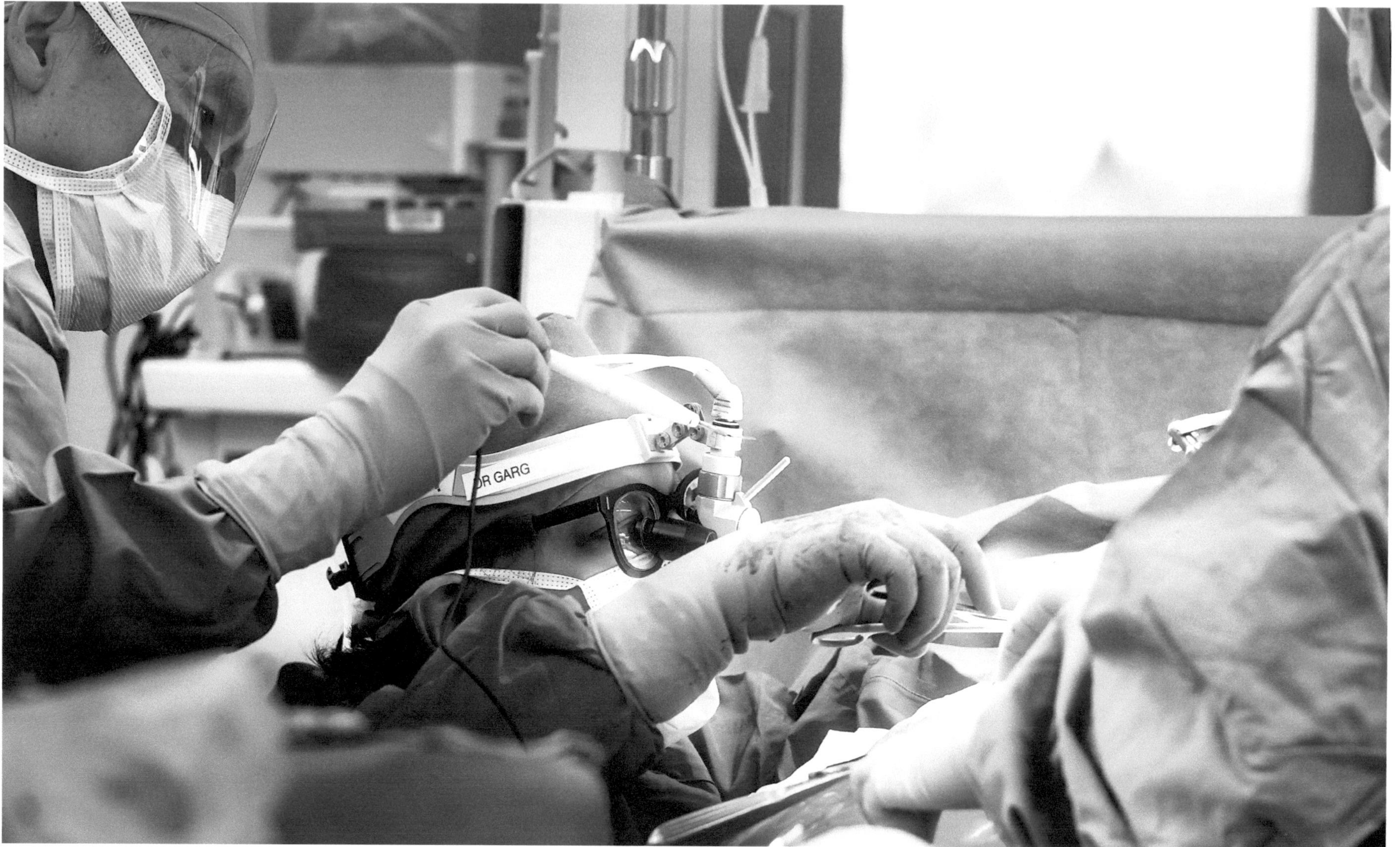

The chest exposed with a retractor in place. Dr. Garg begins taking down the Left Internal Mammary Artery (LIMA) from the chest wall. Patient table is elevated, and Dr. Garg is seated to view the inside undersurface of the left chest

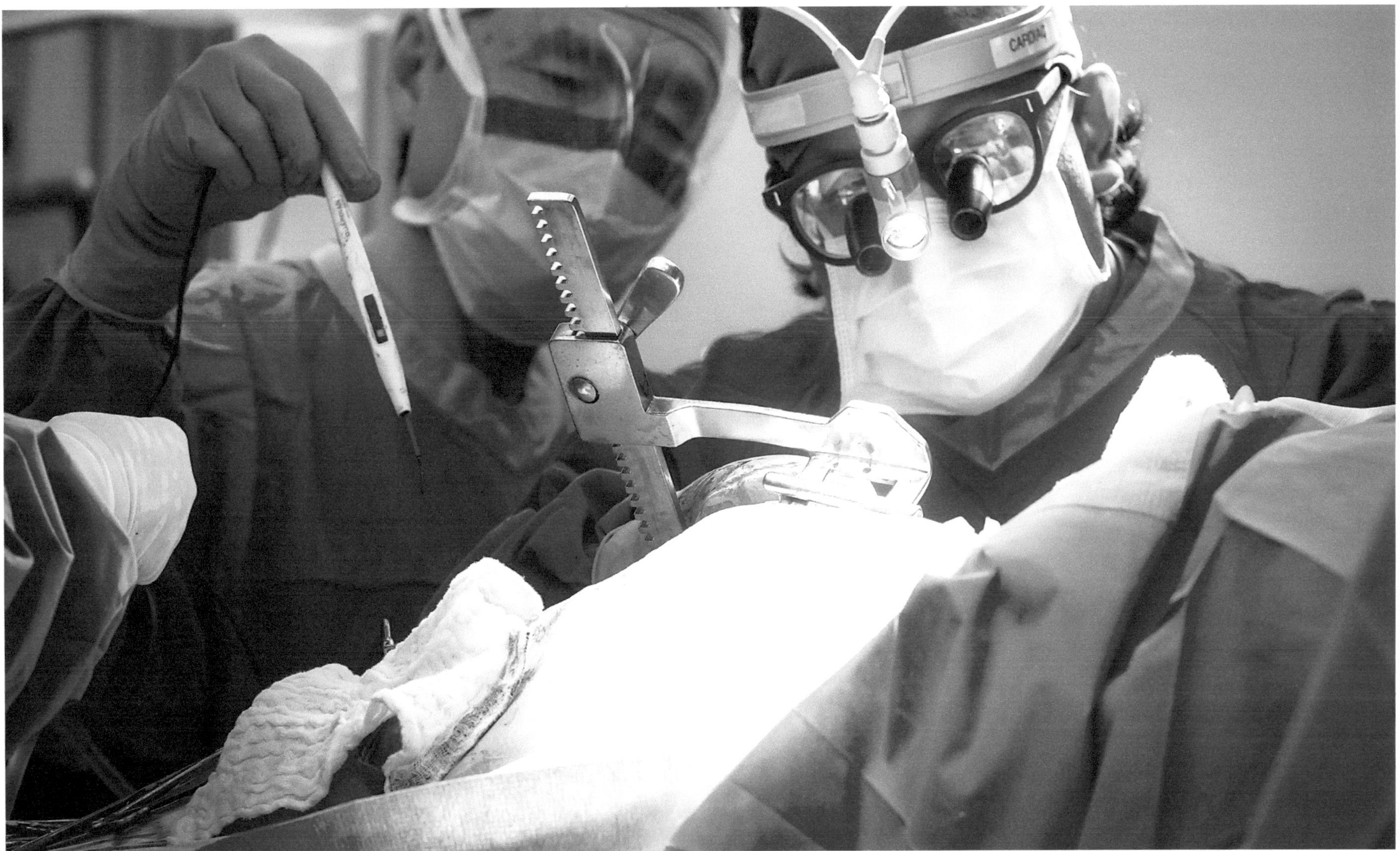

Dr. Garg continues with LIMA dissection from the chest wall with the retractor in place. Second assistant Dr. Chow is holding an electrocautery device for Dr. Garg, a surgical tool he uses for tissue dissection

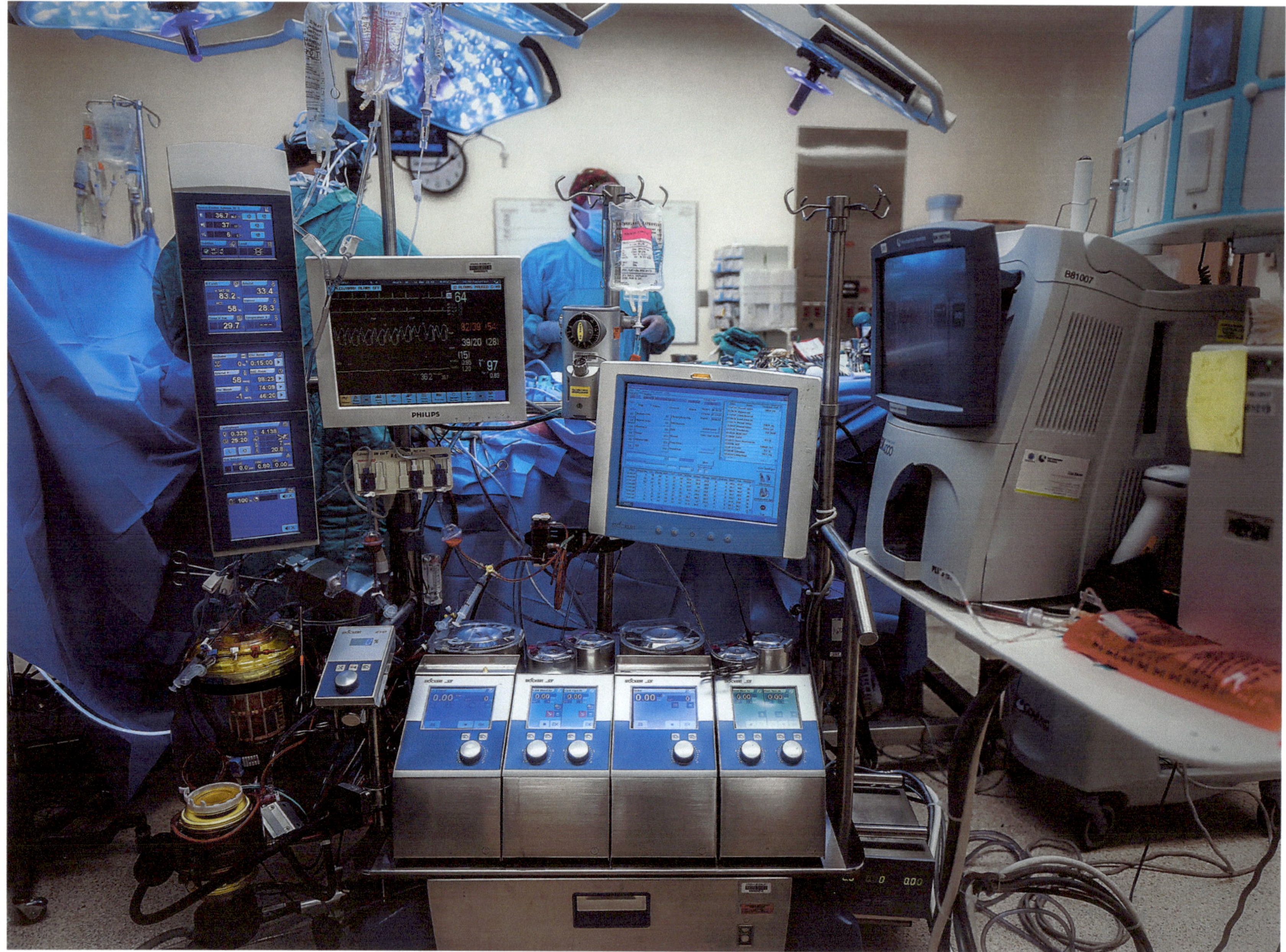

Cardiopulmonary bypass machine

THE HEART LUNG MACHINE
Cardiopulmonary Bypass

As the graft harvesting phase approaches completion, with the left internal mammary artery dissected from the chest and veins harvested from the leg, the next critical phase of the operation begins—to put the patient on the cardiopulmonary bypass (CPB) machine and to arrest the beating heart.

The coronary arteries residing on the heart surface are extraordinarily small in size, typically in the order of 2.0 to 4.0 millimeters in diameter. Due to the small size of coronary arteries and the precision needed to suture harvested grafts to the arteries, a method to operate on a still heart developed in cardiac surgery. This was the cardiopulmonary bypass machine. The machine facilitates cardiac surgery by arresting the heart and lungs, while still maintaining blood flow and oxygenation to the rest of the body.

The development of the cardiopulmonary bypass machine has a fascinating history. In the 1950s, Dr. Walton Lillehei, an American pioneer of cardiac surgery at the University of Minnesota, while operating on an infant to repair a ventricular septal defect (a hole in the heart), used the parent as the bypass machine. In a procedure known as cross-circulation between two individuals, the parent's heart and lungs maintained blood flow and oxygenation during surgery while he operated on the infant. Doubtful critics at the time quoted a 300% mortality with this procedure—the child, the parent, and the surgeon! It marked the nascence of cardiopulmonary bypass in cardiac surgery. Today, the CPB machine is central and routine in the cardiac operating room, with a designated perfusionist running the machine throughout the procedure.

Anticoagulation of the patient is of utmost importance when using this machine. Blood entering and circulating within the machine cannot be allowed to clot. For this reason, the patient is administered with high dose heparin, a blood thinning agent. The two most important parts of this elaborate machine are, the oxygenator and the roller pumps. The oxygenator mimics the lungs, where oxygen-carbon dioxide exchange occurs in the blood. Dark red venous blood from the body is replenished with oxygen, and carbon dioxide is removed to form bright red arterial blood, which is returned to the body. The roller pump imitates the heart function and pumps the blood volume throughout the body. During the time the patient is on the CPB machine, the perfusionist carefully manages numerous statistics, including oxygenation, blood flow, blood-thinning adequacy, electrolyte levels, arterial pressure, core temperature, arterial and venous blood gases, and blood volume status.

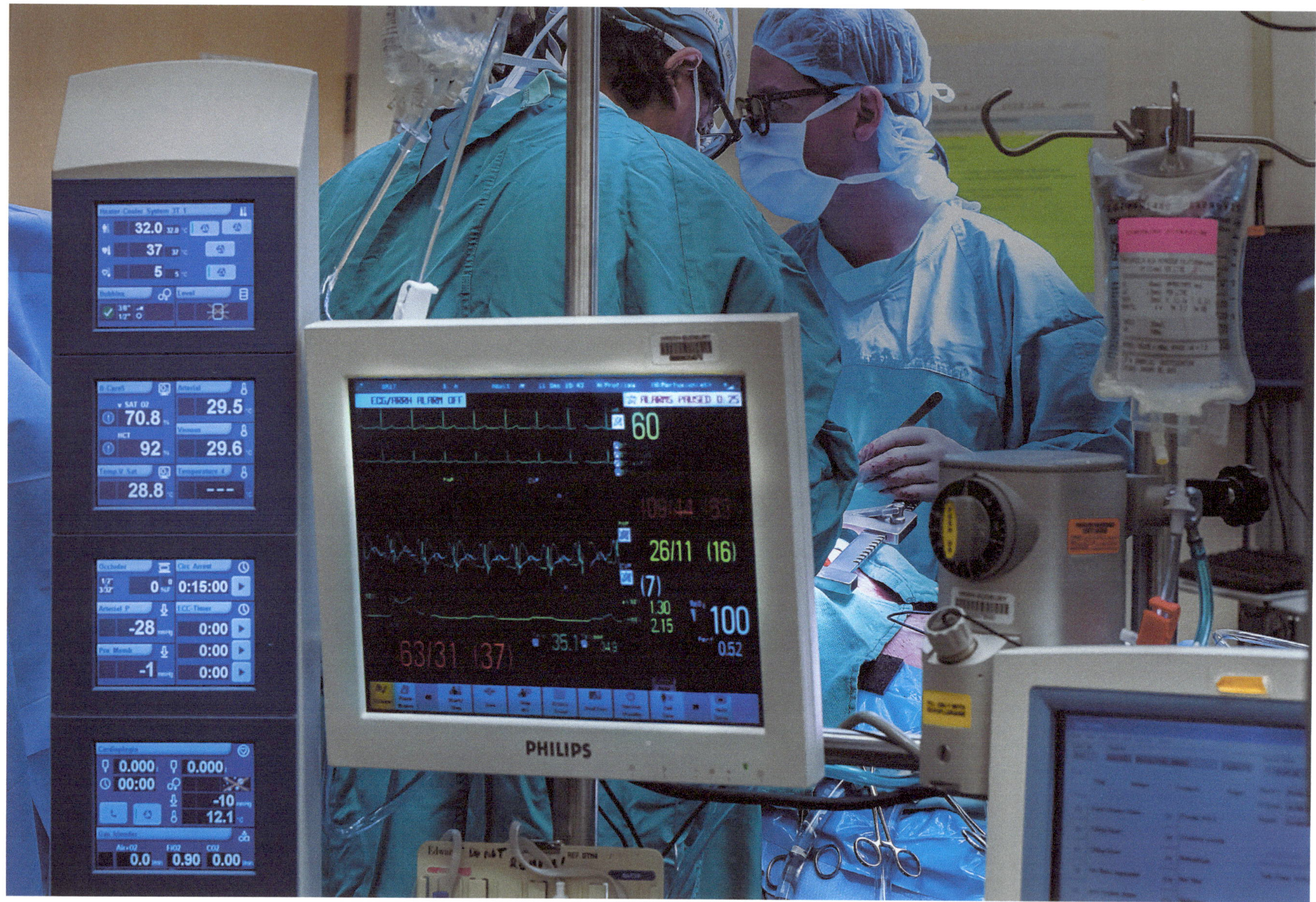

Close up of the CPB machine monitor showing the patient's heart beat at 60 beats per minute

With the grafts harvested, the patient is put on the CPB machine by the surgeon, following intravenous heparinization. Venous and arterial cannulas are connected to the CPB machine. The arterial cannula is inserted into the ascending aorta, and the venous cannula is inserted into the right atrium. The patient's body temperature is cooled to 32 degrees Celsius.

The next phase is arresting the heart. The surgeon does this by first clamping the aorta to isolate the heart from the rest of the body's circulatory system. This prevents blood circulation to the coronary arteries. In order to preserve the heart and stop it from beating, the surgeon inserts a small catheter (also known as the cardioplegia line) into the aorta from the CPB machine, and flushes a cold (4 degrees Celsius) high potassium blood solution into the heart. The high potassium arrests the heart, the cold temperature reduces it's metabolic needs, while the blood solution provides it with oxygen and nutrients.

In following chapters, I have chosen to exhibit color photographs in order to identify arterial and venous components of the cardiopulmonary bypass circuit. Patient is "on pump," and the heart is arrested.

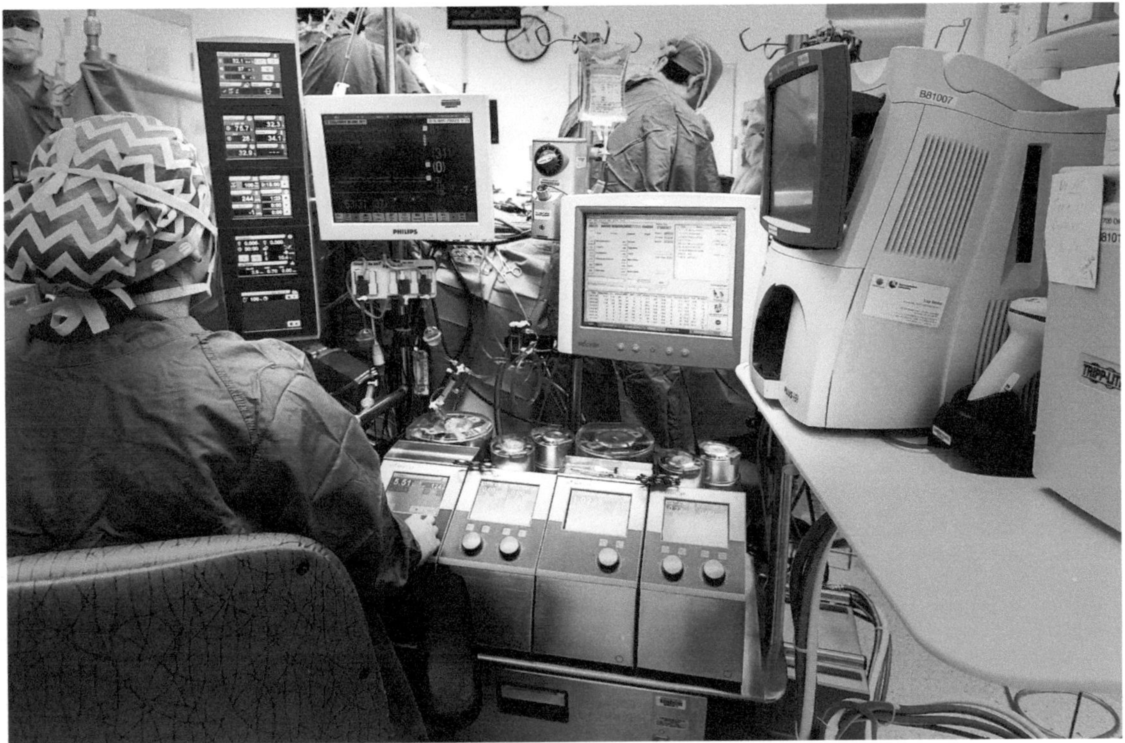

Perfusionist monitoring stats on CPB machine while patient is on cardiopulmonary bypass

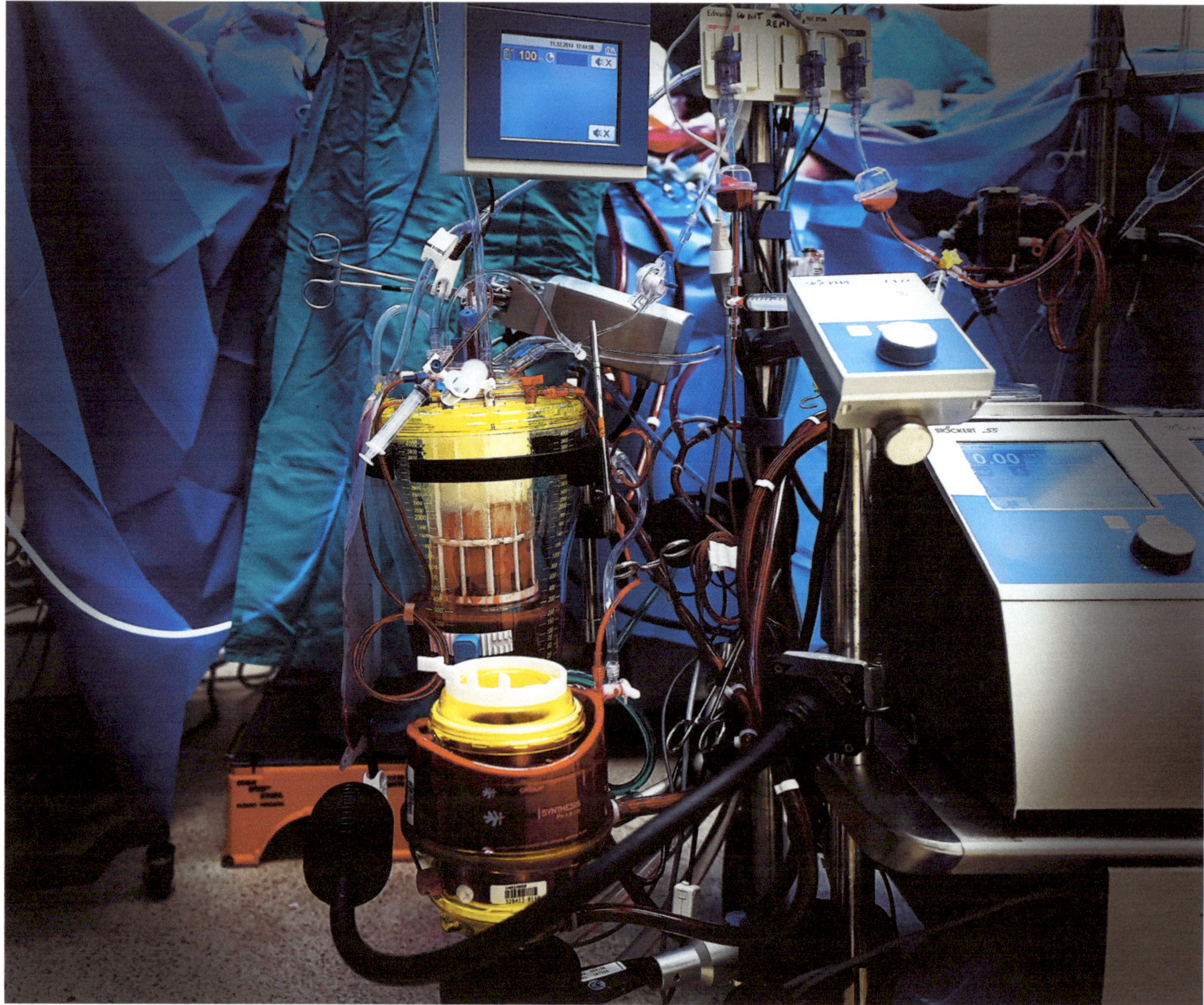

Blood oxygenator of the CPB machine

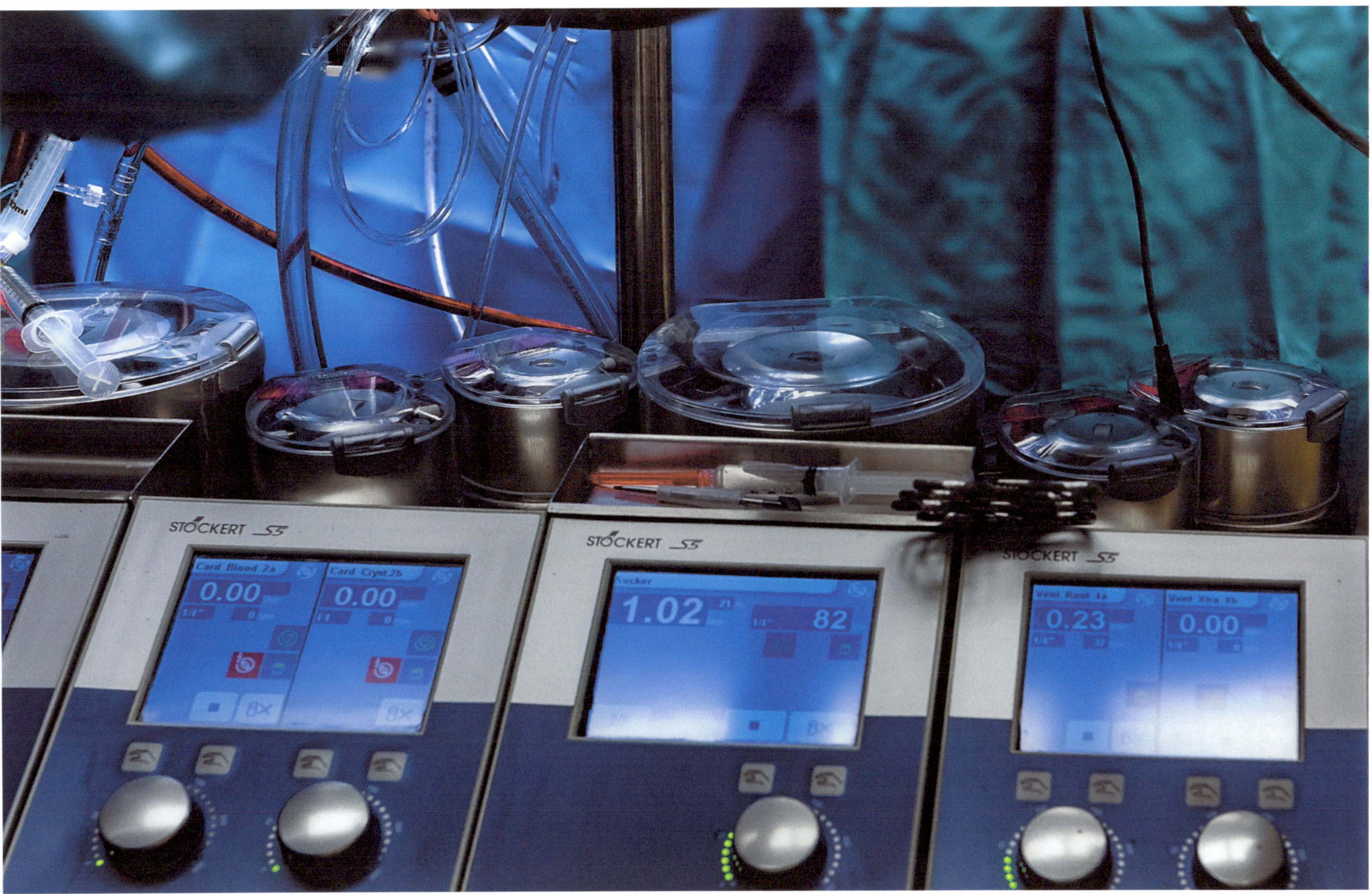

Roller pumps of the CPB machine

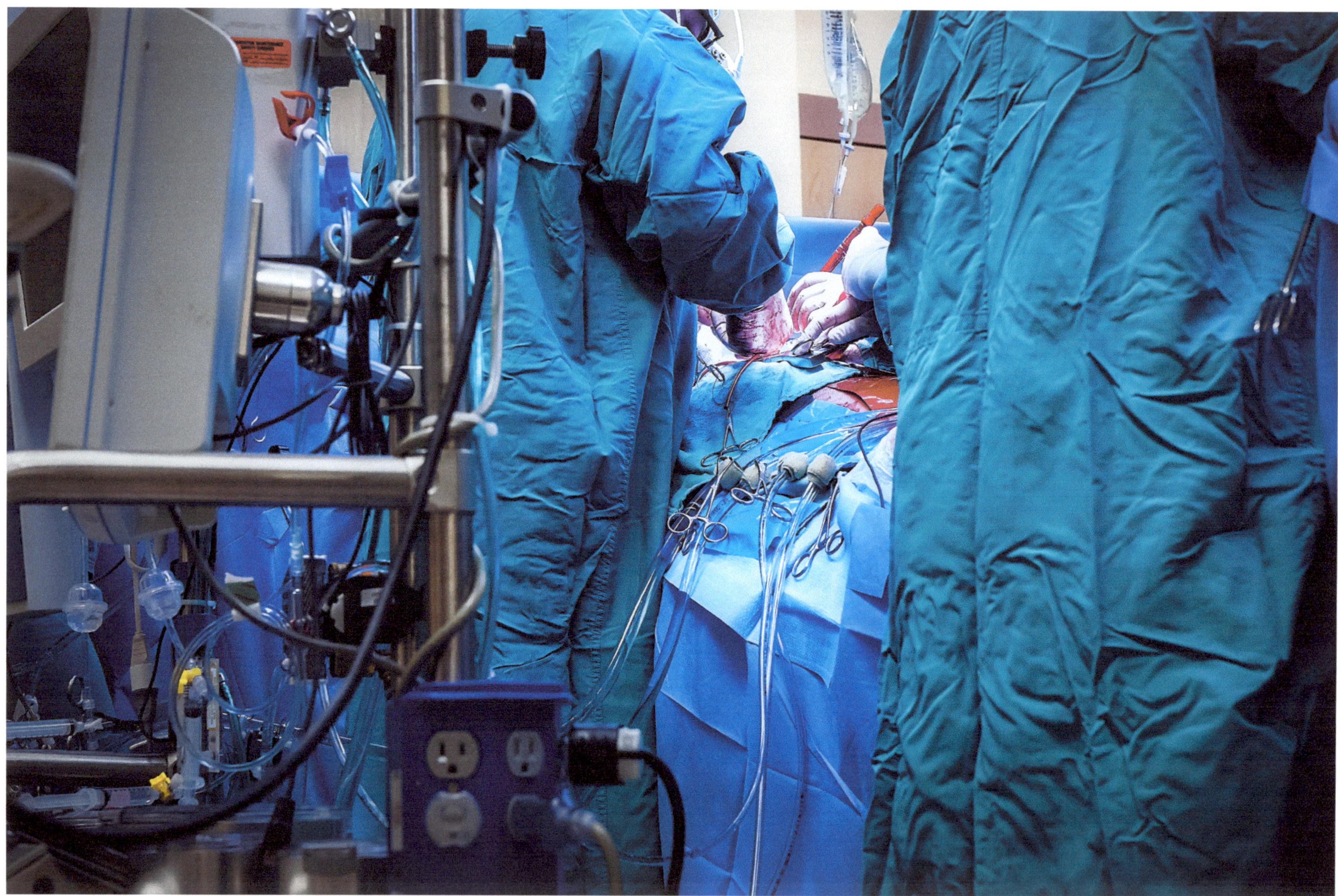

Placement of arterial and venous cannulas to establish the CPB circuit

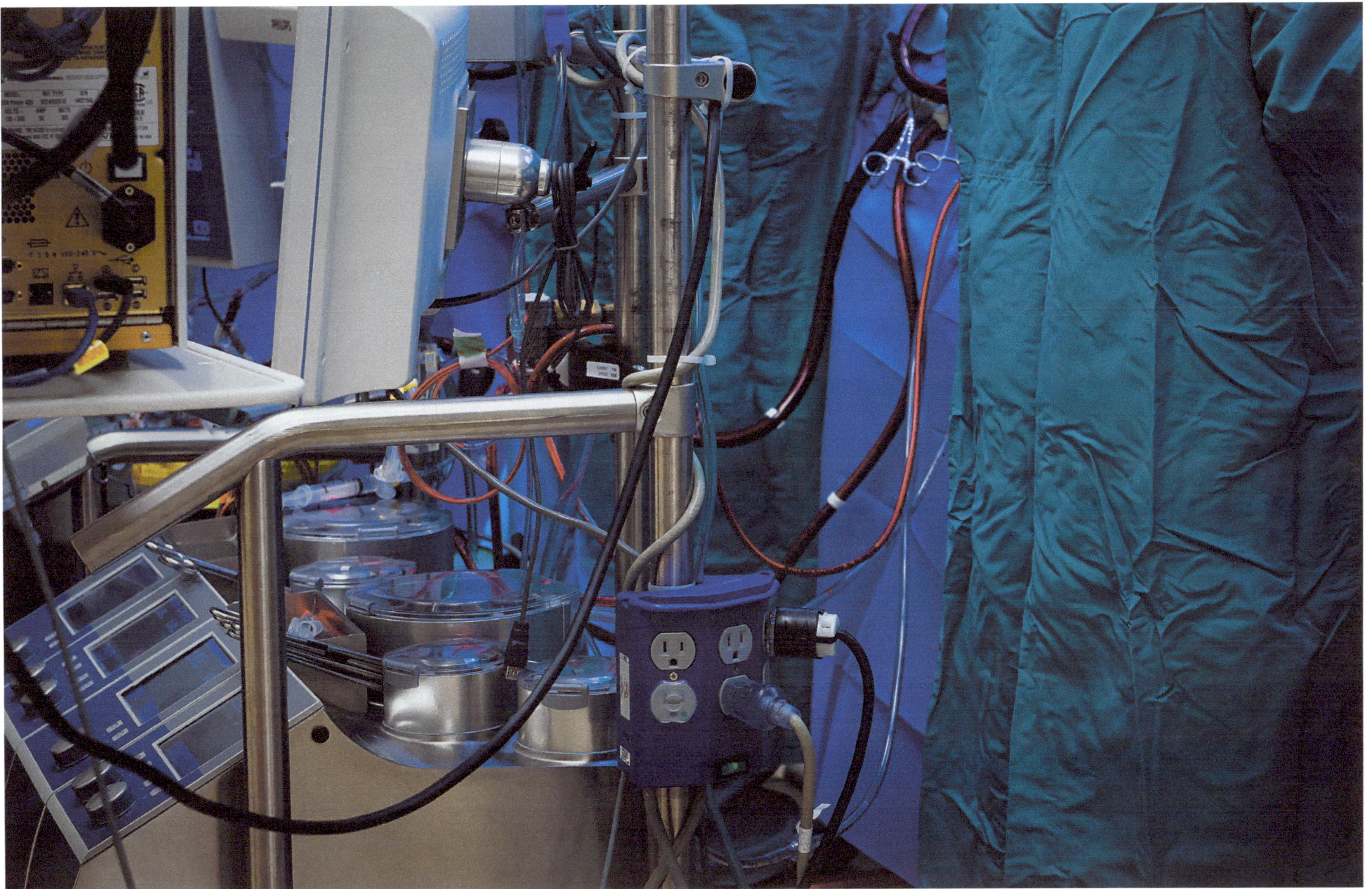

Patient is "on pump". Venous blood is in the cannula carrying dark red blood going from the patient to the CPB machine, while the bright red blood is oxygenated arterial blood from the machine back to the patient.

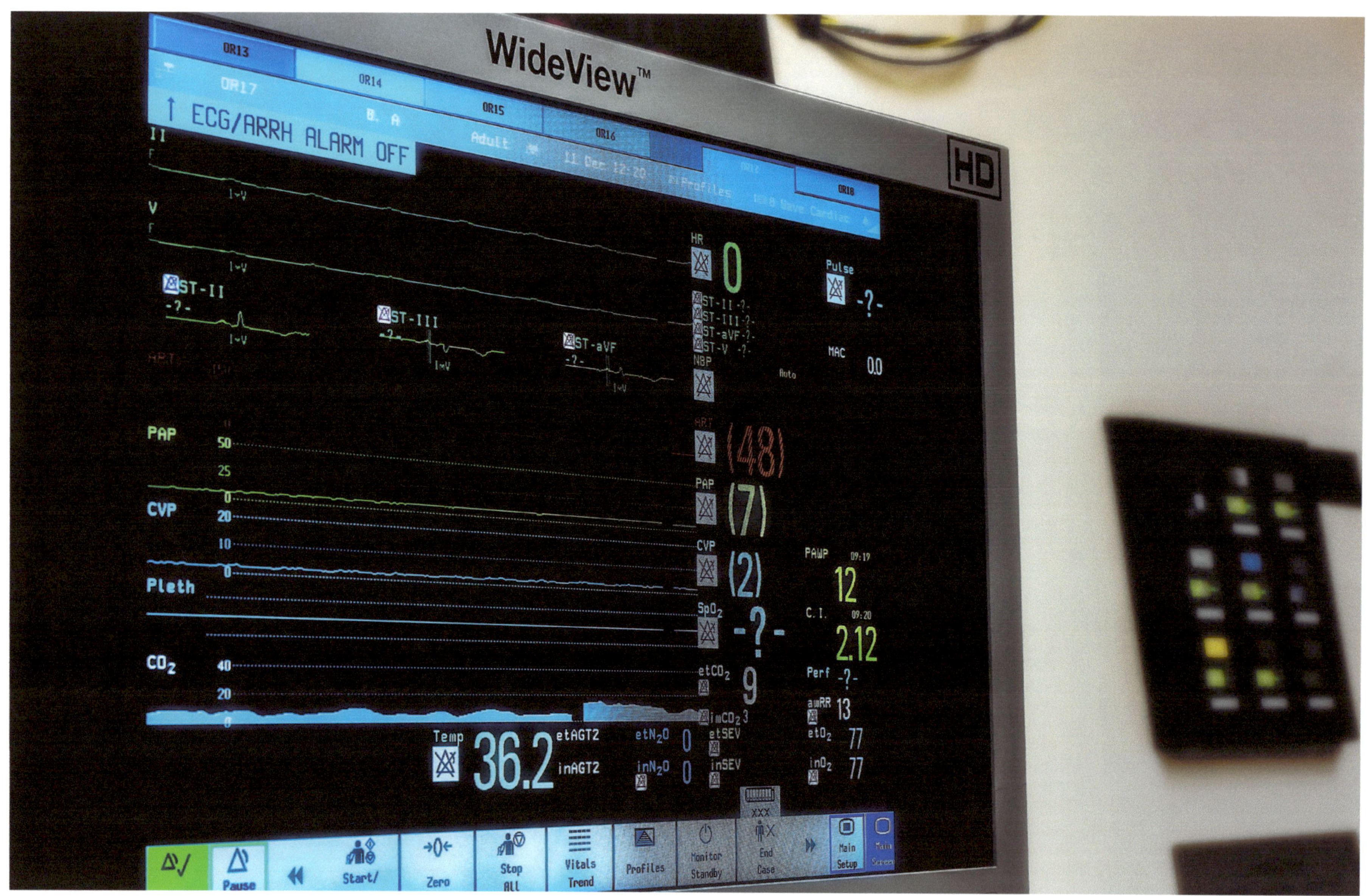

Aortic cross-clamp in place and cardioplegia administered. Heart has arrested—no heart beat and flat line on ECG

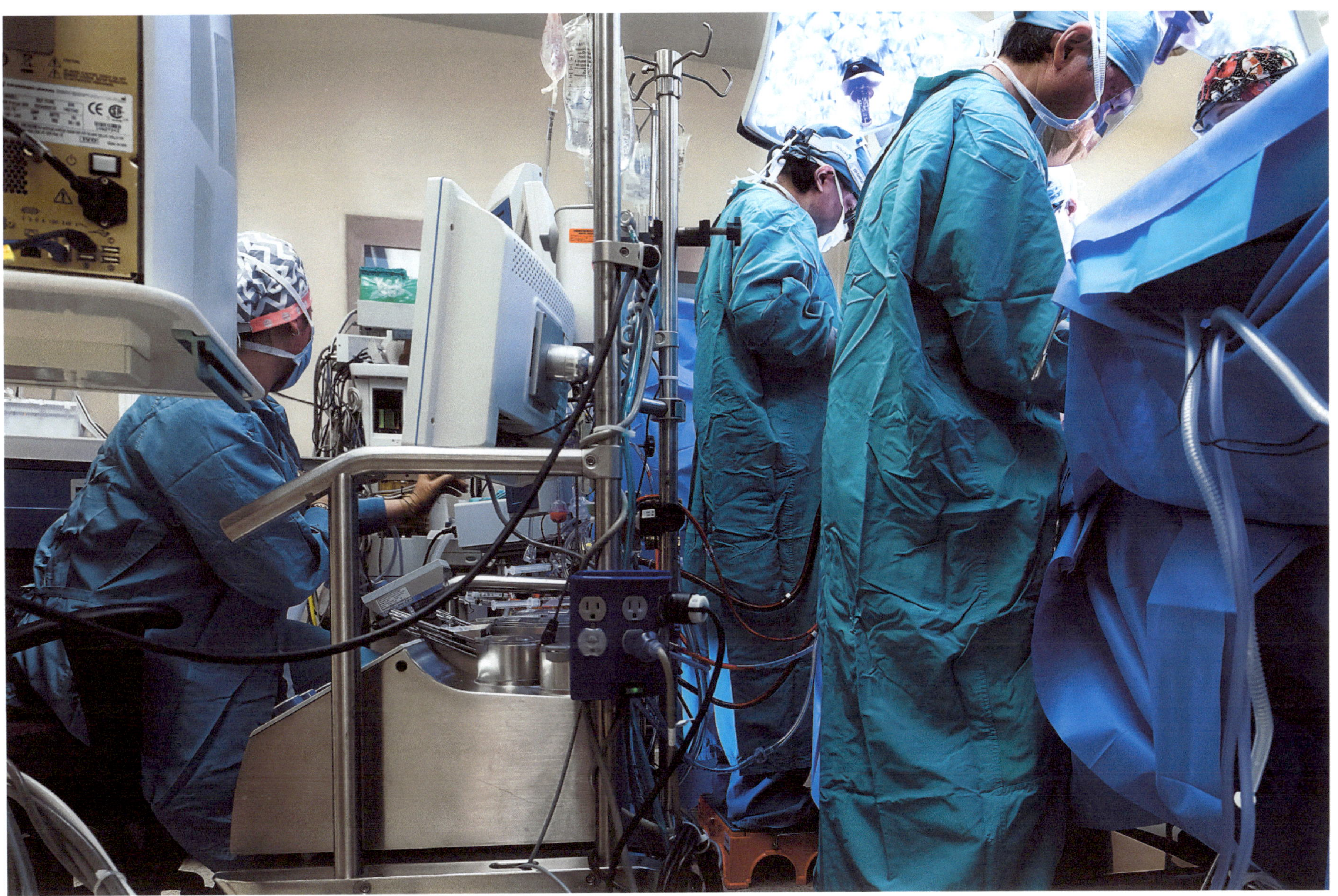

With patient on Cardiopulmonary Bypass, coronary artery bypass grafting underway

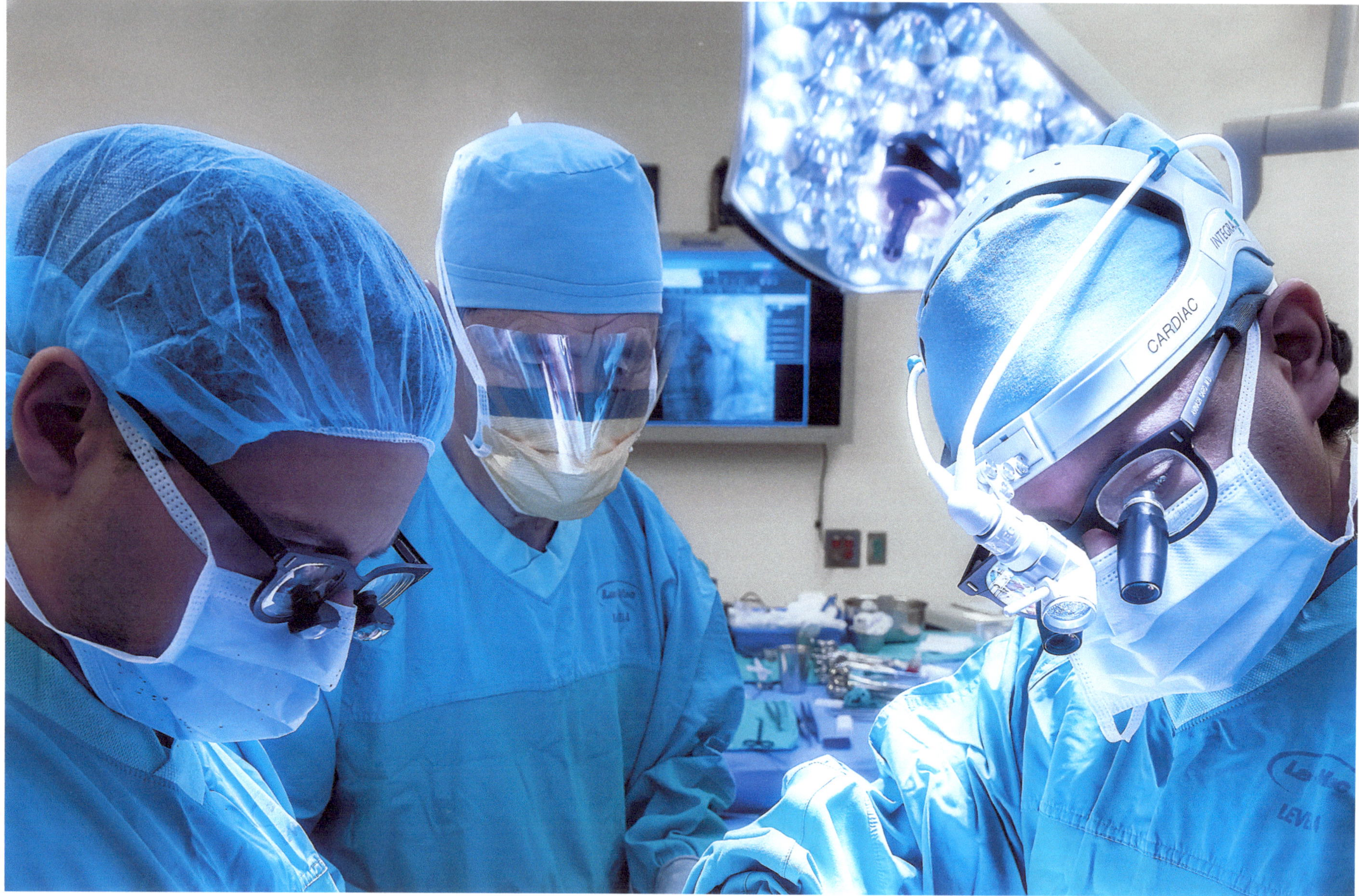

Right: Lead surgeon Dr. Garg; Left: First Assistant Dr. Atoui; Middle: Second Assistant Dr. Chow

CORONARY ARTERY BYPASS GRAFTING

With the patient on cardiopulmonary bypass, the body is cooled to 32 degree Celsius to reduce its metabolic needs. With veins and LIMA (left internal mammary artery) harvested, coronary artery bypass grafting now begins.

The two main coronary arteries supplying blood to the heart are, the left main coronary artery and the right coronary artery (RCA). The right coronary artery supplies blood to approximately one third of the heart. The left main coronary artery bifurcates into two arteries, the left anterior descending (LAD) and the circumflex coronary artery and supplies blood to the remaining two-thirds of the heart. Left main stem (LMS) occlusion before the bifurcation is especially critical because it results in death with no chance of survival, since blood flow is blocked to two-thirds of the heart—incompatible with life. Left main stem disease is often referred to as the "widow maker." It is treated by creating bypasses to both branches of the LMS, the LAD and the circumflex coronary arteries.

This patient is a sixty-two-year-old gentleman who presented with increasing chest pain with a strongly positive exercise stress test. The coronary angiogram showed the patient had a 90% stenosis, or blockage, in the left main stem. The LAD, circumflex, and RCA had no disease, with normal left ventricular function. Ventricular function describes the contractility of the heart, or its ability to pump.

In this case, the patient underwent triple bypass surgery, with bypasses to both branches of the left main stem. He received an arterial LIMA graft to the LAD and a vein graft to the circumflex coronary artery. He also received an additional vein graft to a branch of the LAD.

As mentioned earlier, at this stage, the patient is on cardiopulmonary bypass, the aorta is clamped, the heart has arrested, and the surgeon proceeds to create the necessary bypasses. In the photographs that follow, we see the surgeon creating new paths using the harvested venous and arterial grafts to divert blood flow, thereby circumventing the blockages.

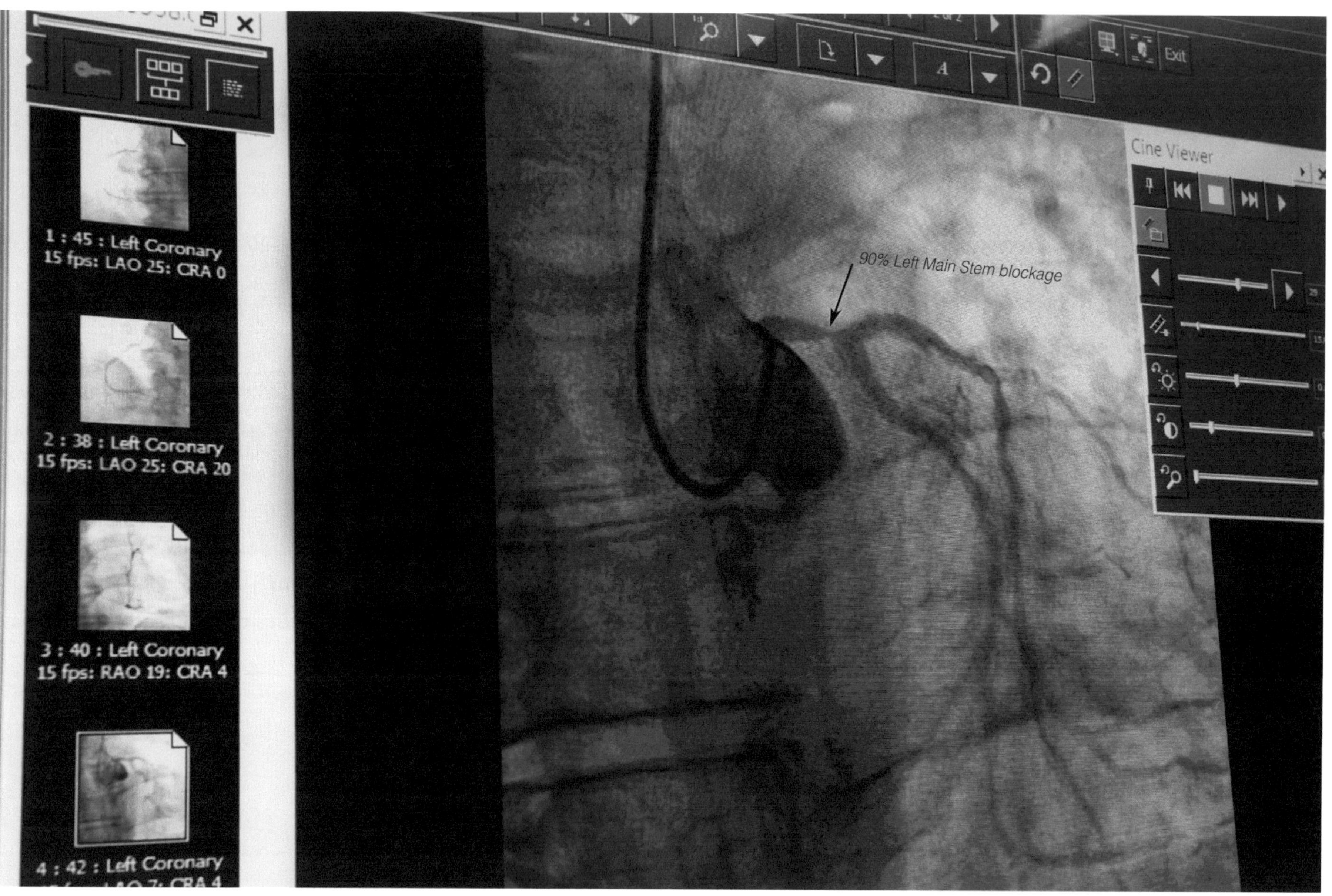

Patient's coronary angiogram on the display monitor in the operating room. Visible is the sharp narrowing of the LMS showing the 90% blockage just before it bifurcates into the LAD and circumflex coronary arteries.

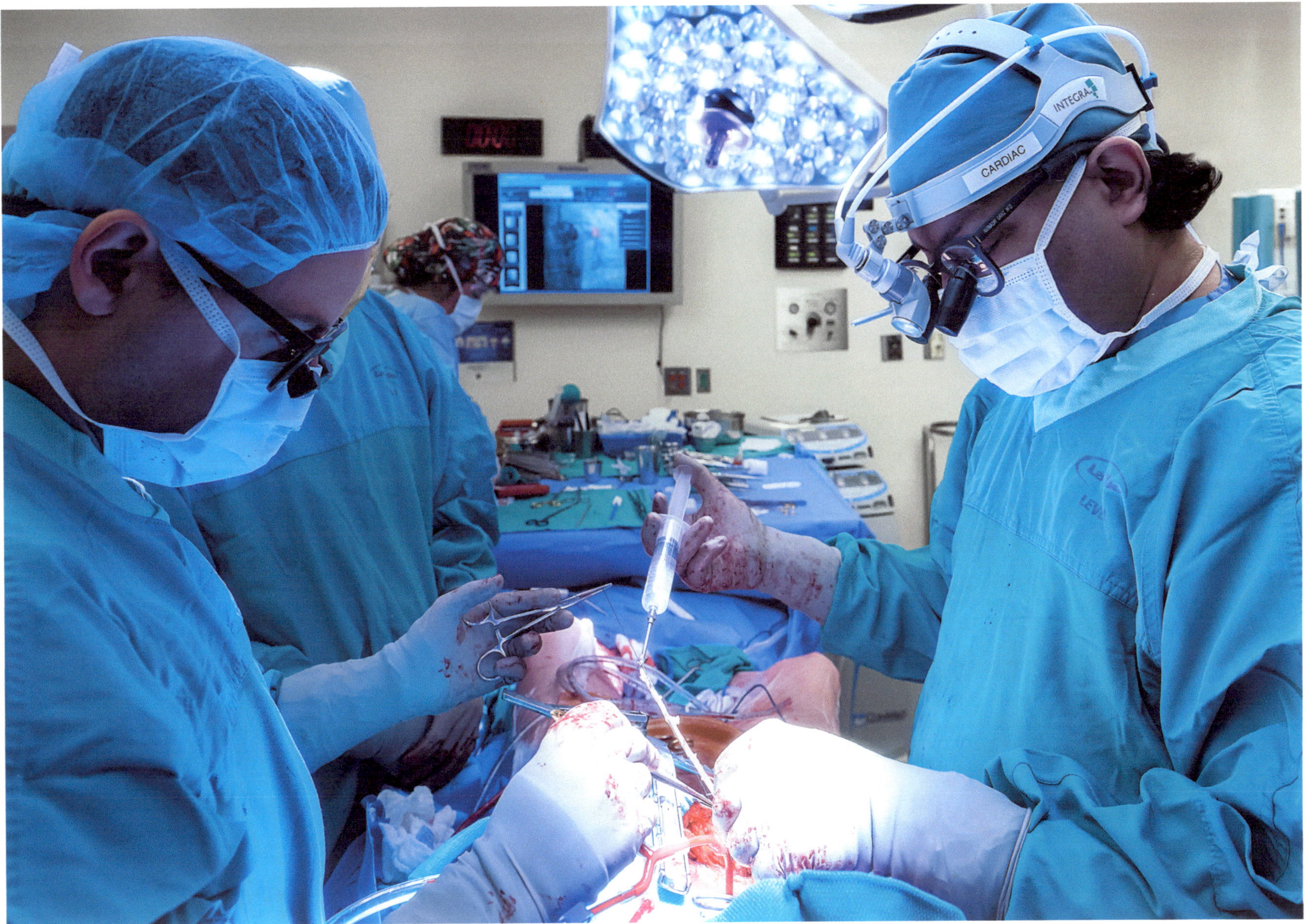

Harvested vein graft from the leg is examined for length and integrity

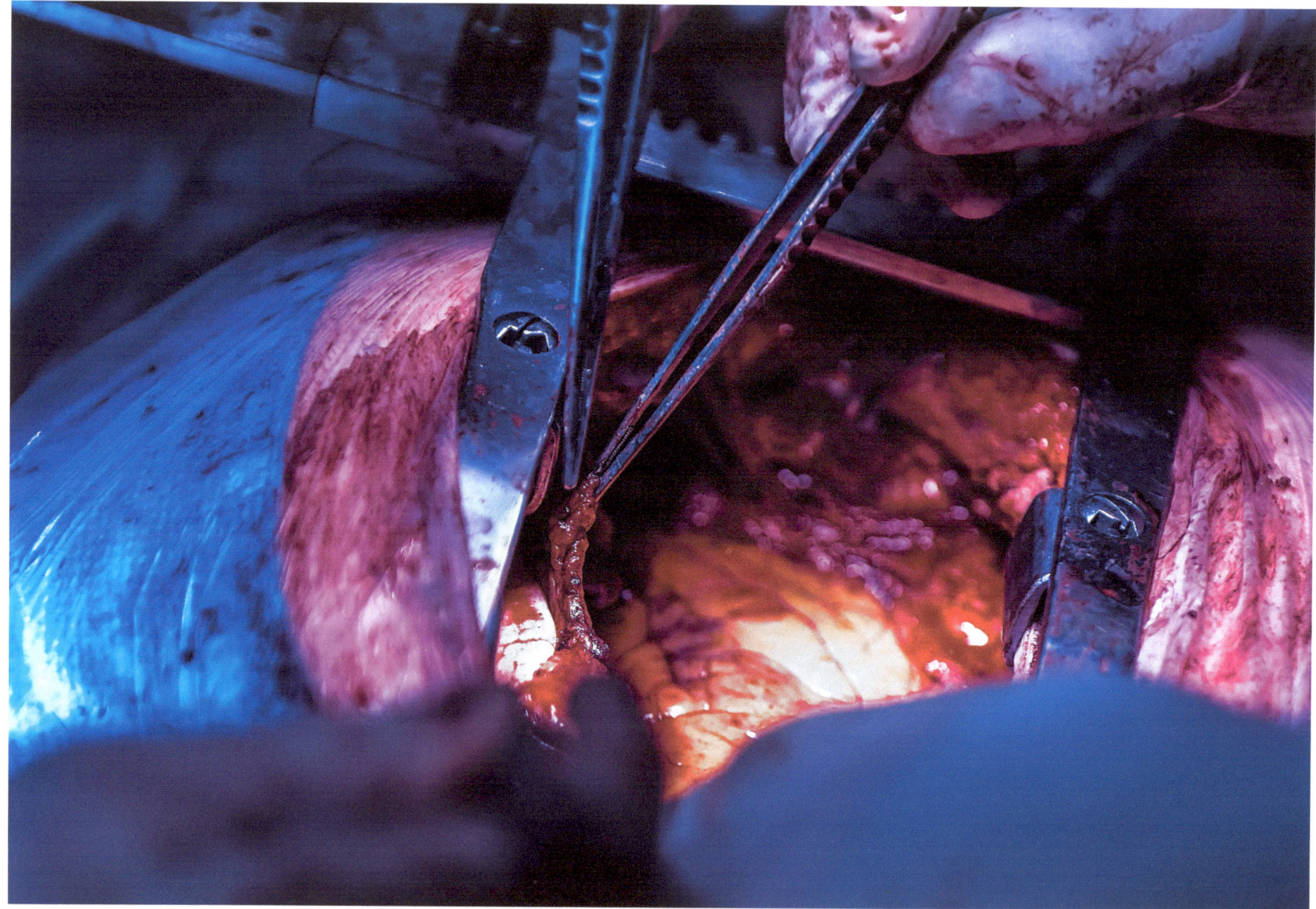

Harvested left internal mammary artery from undersurface of the chest—to be used for the arterial graft

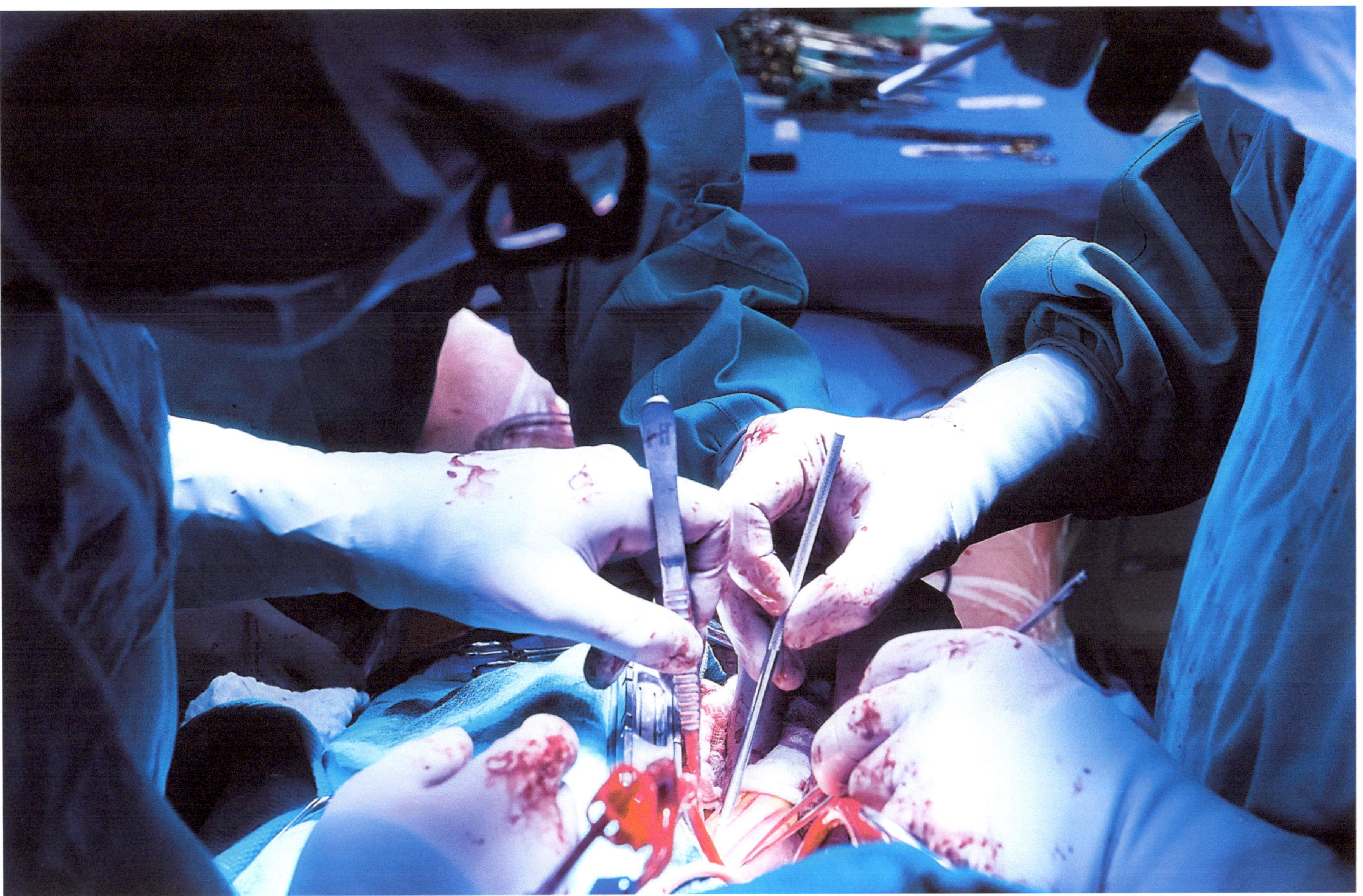

Heart exposed, LAD coronary artery dissection in progress

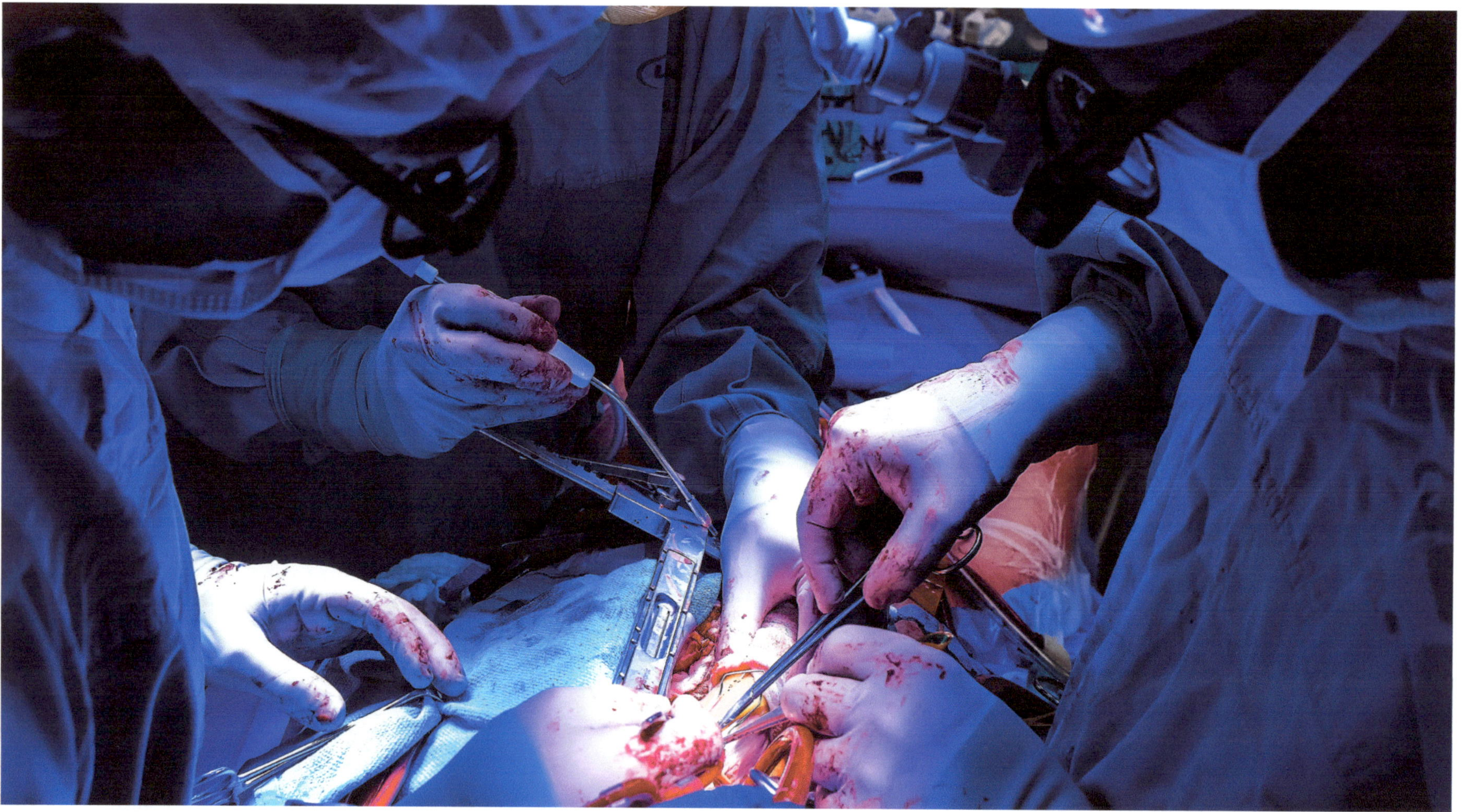

With the LAD opened at the determined site, the terminal end of the LIMA graft is being sutured to the artery, in surgical terms—the distal LIMA coronary anastomosis

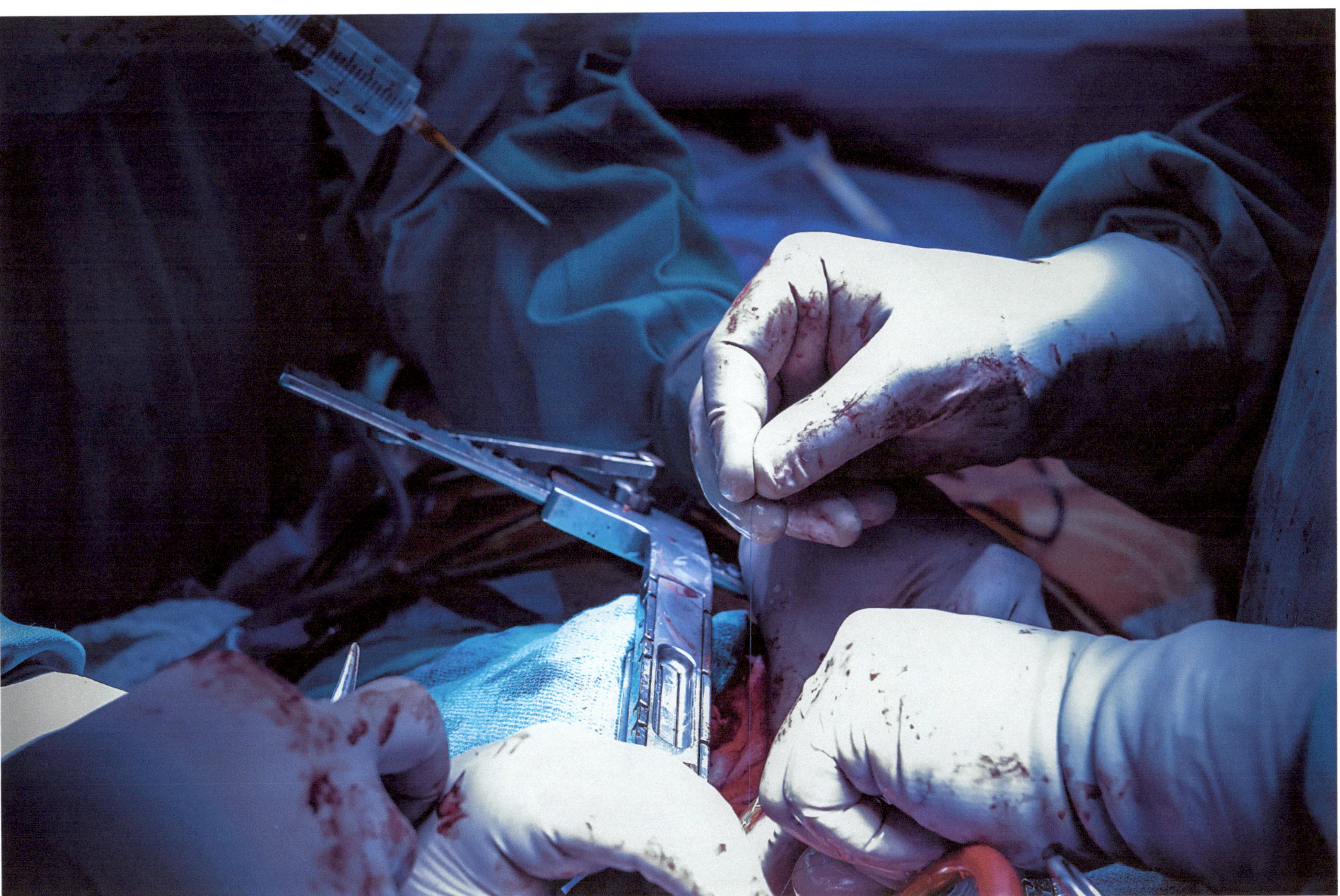

Suture is tightened with terminal end of LIMA graft secured in position to the LAD

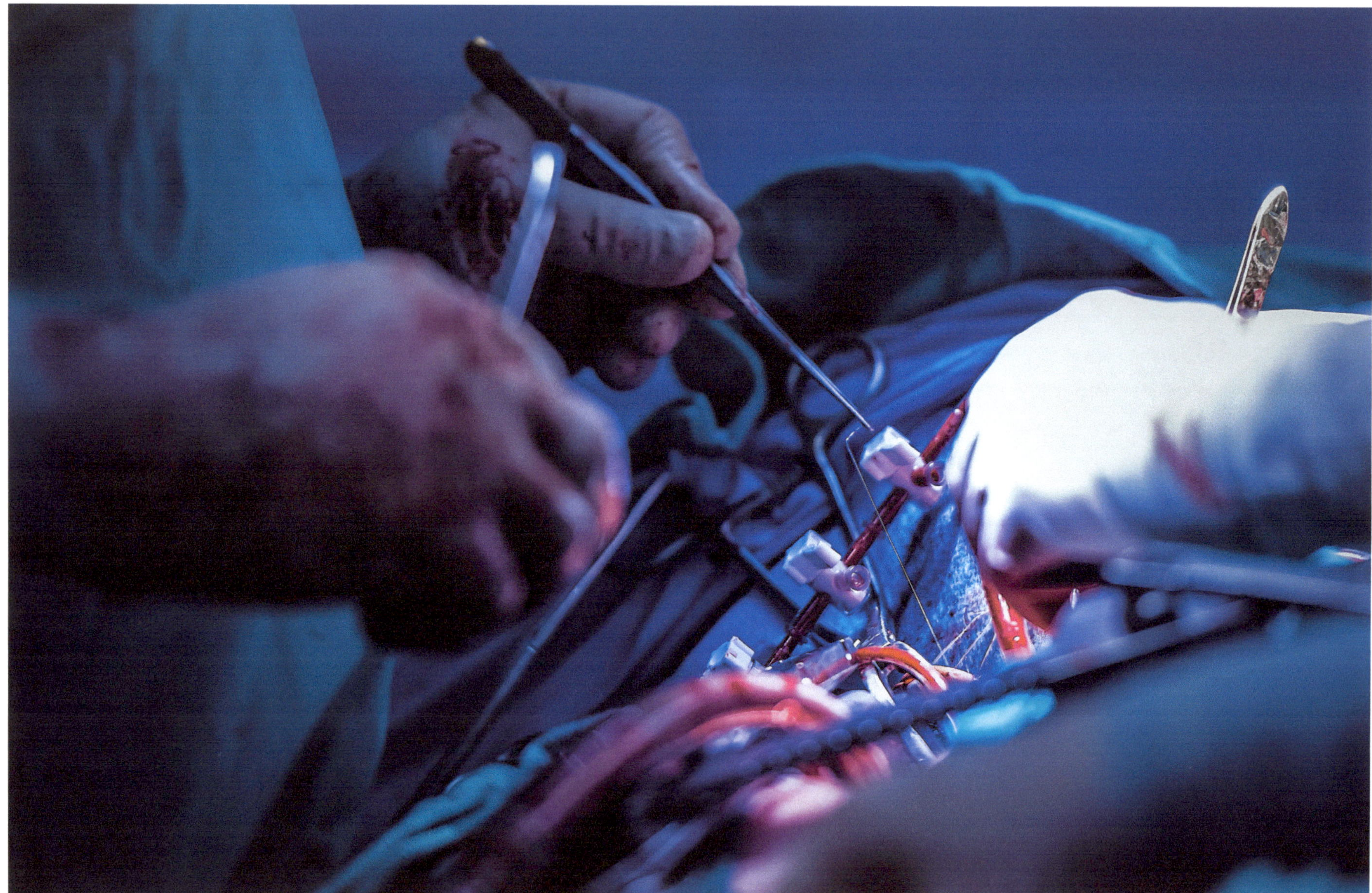

Suturing process continues

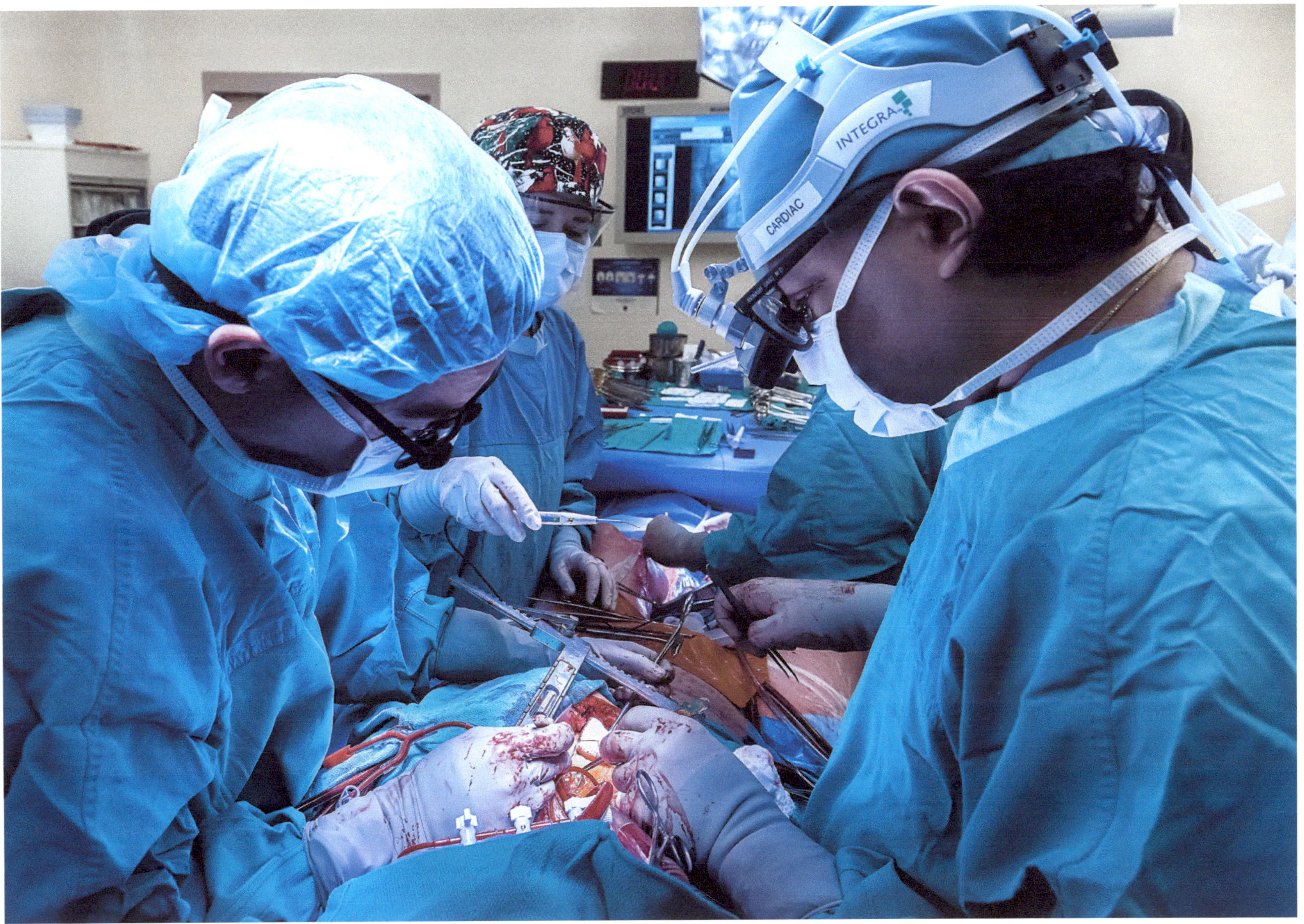

Completion of LIMA graft

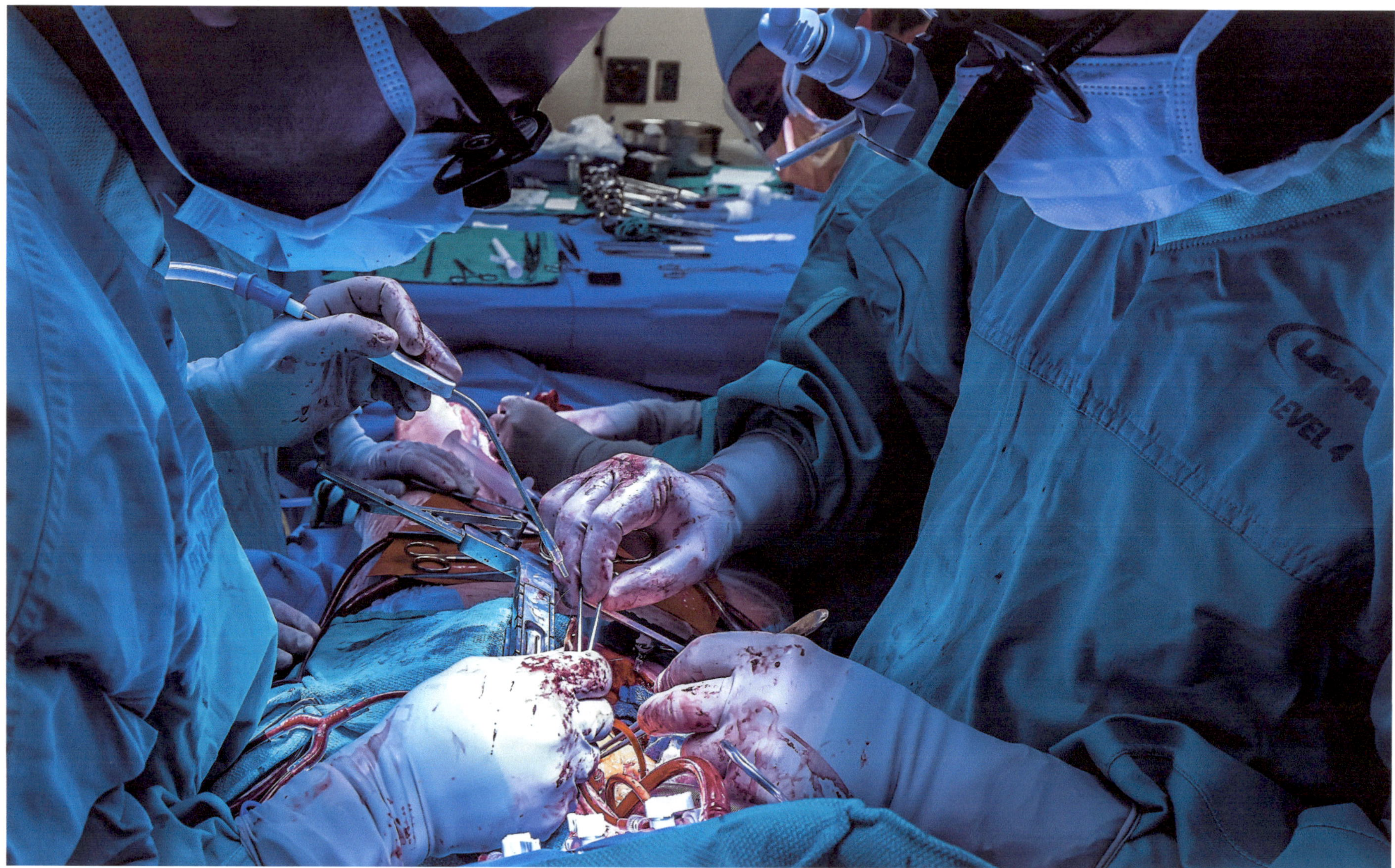

Suturing of other vein grafts continues

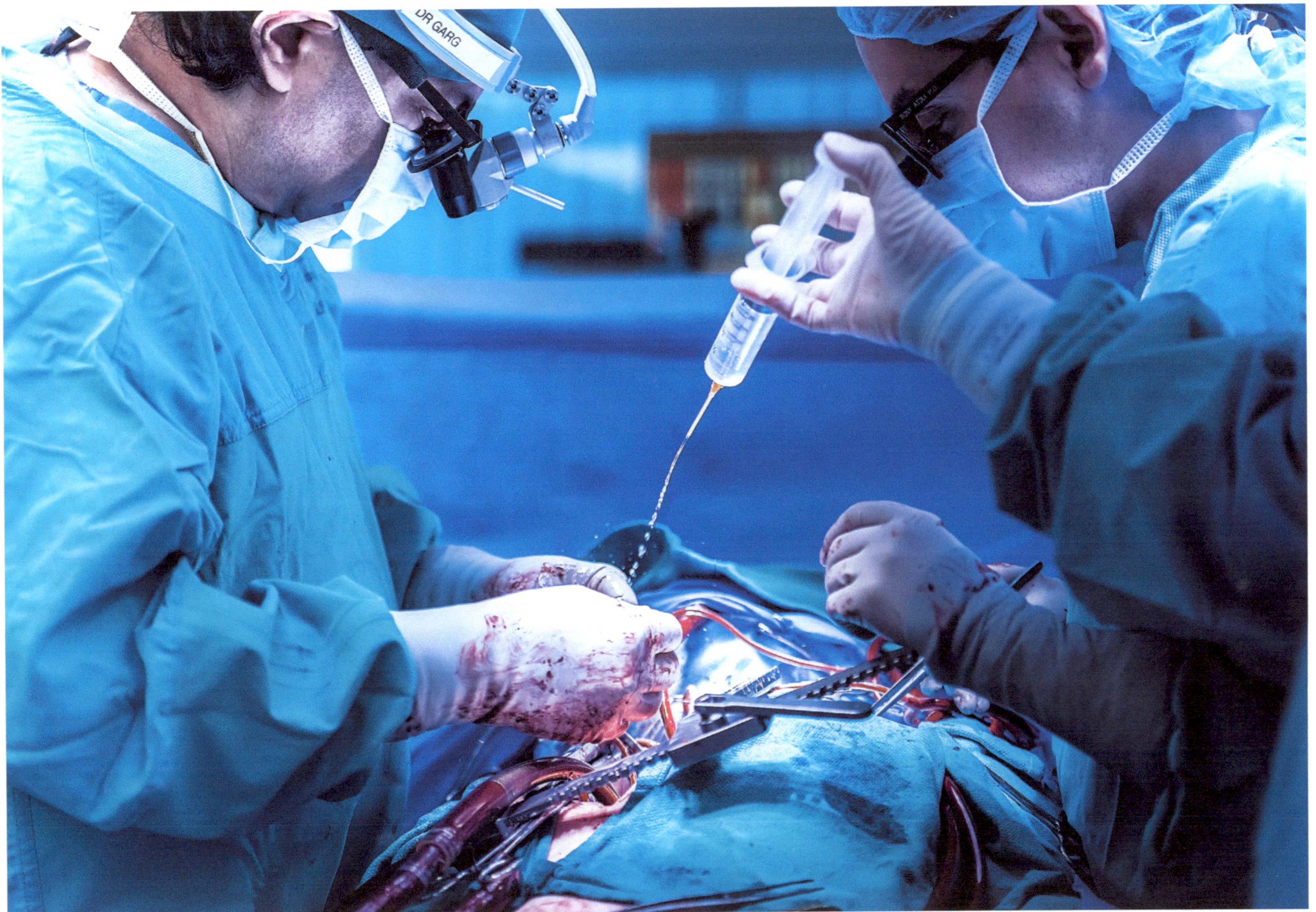

The surgeon's hands drenched with saline solution to provide a frictionless surface on the gloves, making it easier for the super-fine sutures to slide over the fingers during the suturing process

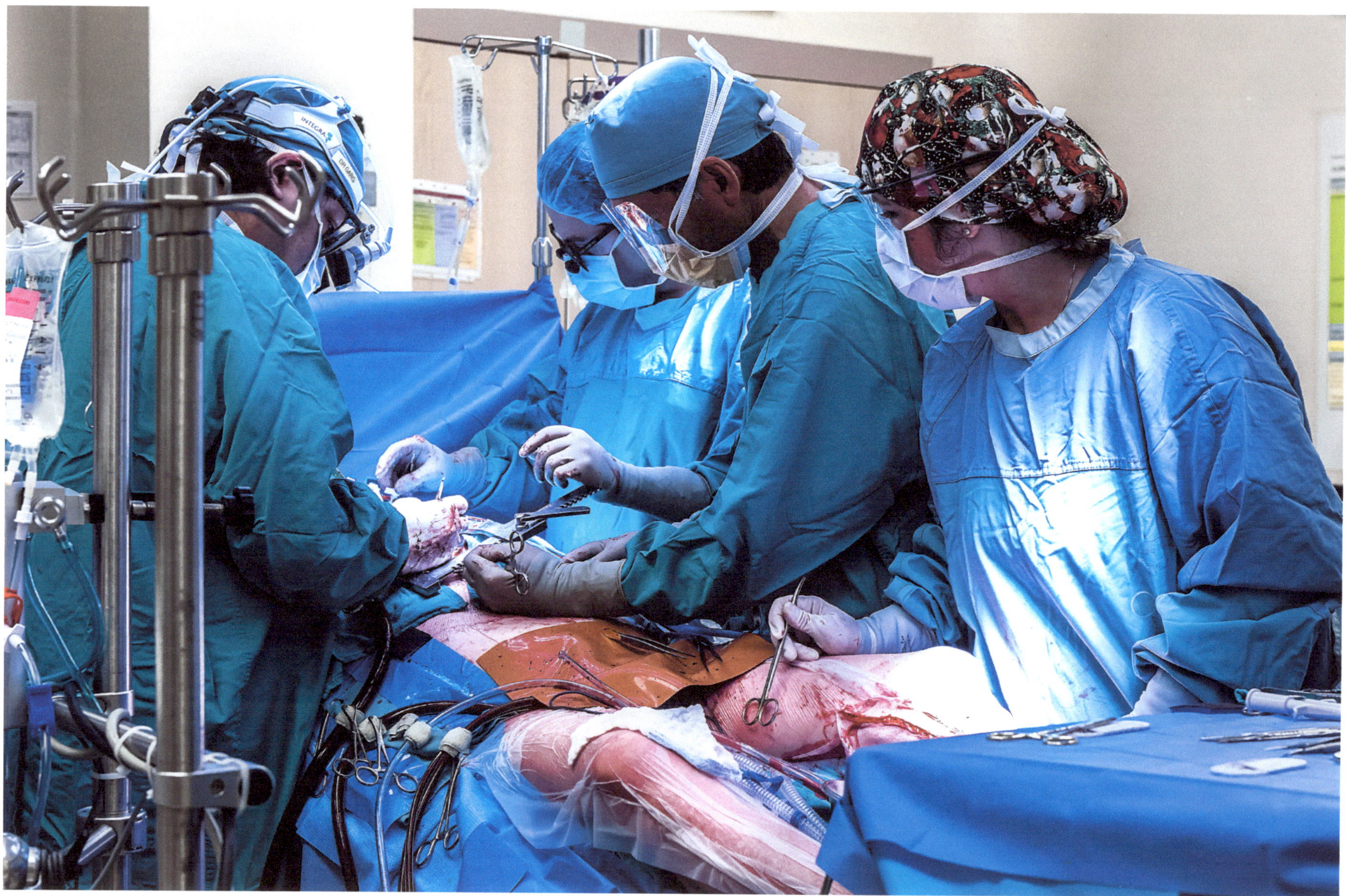

Grafting continues

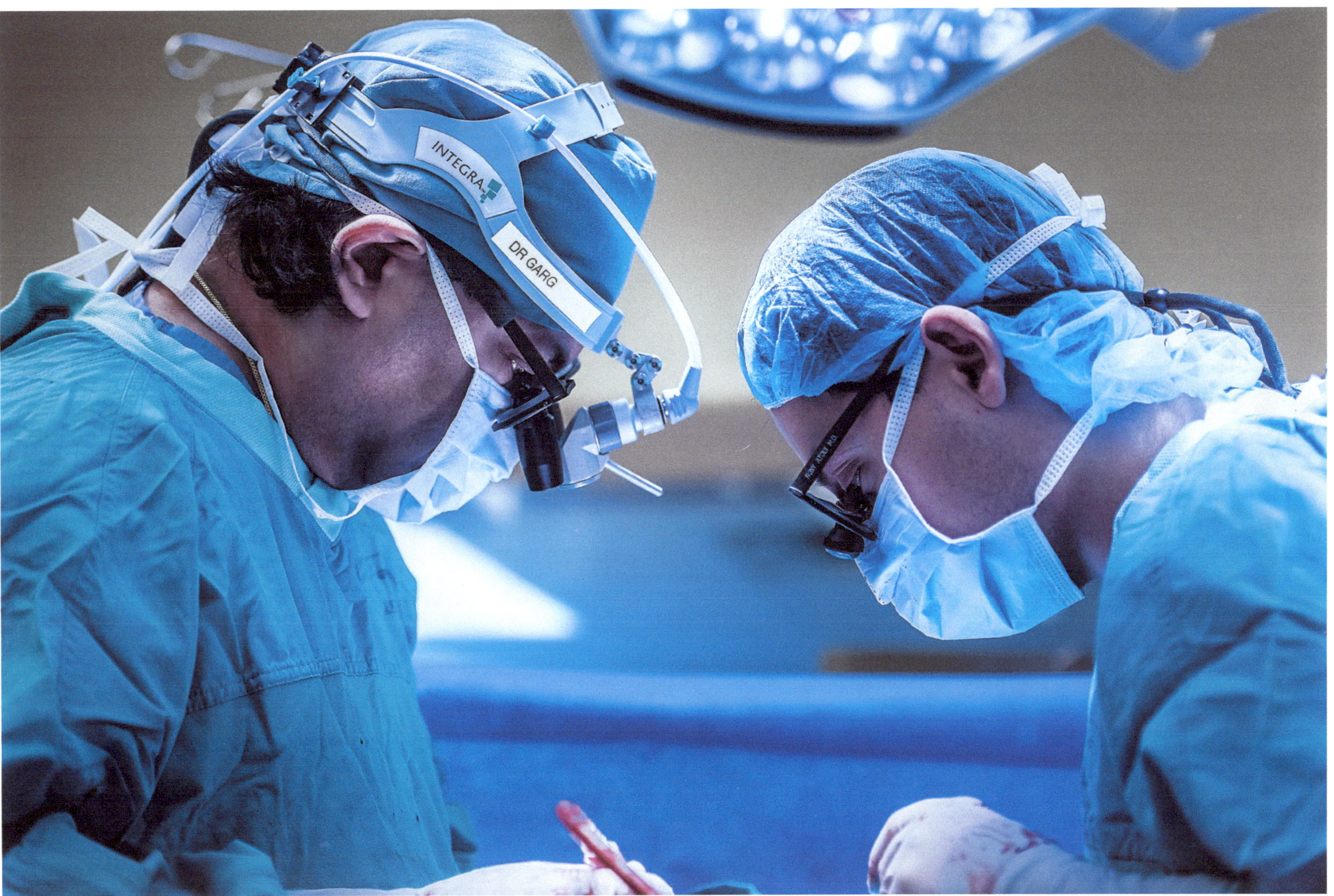

Left: Cardiac Surgeon Dr. Avinash Garg; Right: Cardiac Surgeon Dr. Rony Atoui

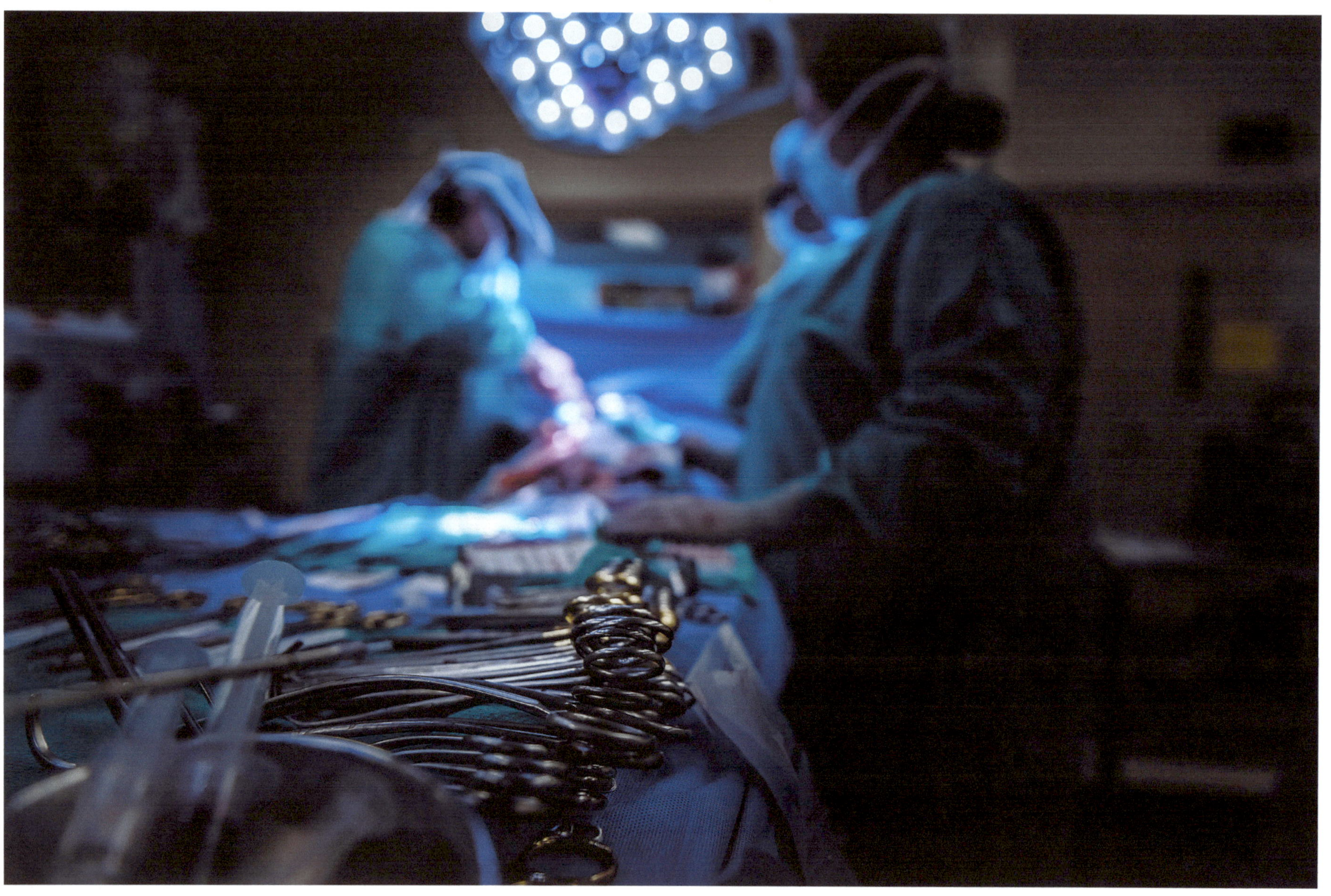

Weaning From Cardiopulmonary Bypass & Chest Closure

At this stage of the operation, coronary artery bypass grafting is complete. The surgeon has created the necessary coronary bypasses using the left internal mammary artery and vein grafts. The next phase is to get the rehabilitated heart beating again, with its newly constructed blood supply system. To recall, the patient was administered with anti-coagulation, placed on cardiopulmonary bypass, cooled to 32 degrees Celsius and then the heart was arrested. These series of processes must be reversed, as the patient is weaned off the CPB machine and the heart resumes its own ability to pump.

The first phase begins with the surgeon indicating to the perfusionist that the patient is ready to come off pump. At this point, there is visible activity again in the operating room, the anesthetist has returned, and the perfusionist is actively monitoring patient statistics. Clearly there is a break in tension from about an hour of intense concentration of the entire team during the process of coronary grafting.

The perfusionist begins to gradually rewarm the patient back to 36.5 degrees Celsius by way of a heat exchanger in the CPB machine, which slowly warms the circulating blood volume. In order to "awaken" the arrested heart, the surgeon flushes the heart with 500 milliliters of warm blood (36 degrees Celsius), often referred to as the "hot shot," through the cardioplegia line previously inserted to arrest the heart. Firstly, this enables the heart to rewarm from 4 degrees Celsius, and secondly, it helps to flush out the high potassium solution that was administered to arrest the heart for the grafting process. Typically, the heart responds spontaneously and begins beating in normal sinus rhythm. This is quite an impressive moment in the operating room, with all eyes watching the ECG monitor as it goes from displaying a flat-line zero heart rhythm to spontaneously displaying signs of rhythm and life. This patient's heart began beating in sinus rhythm.

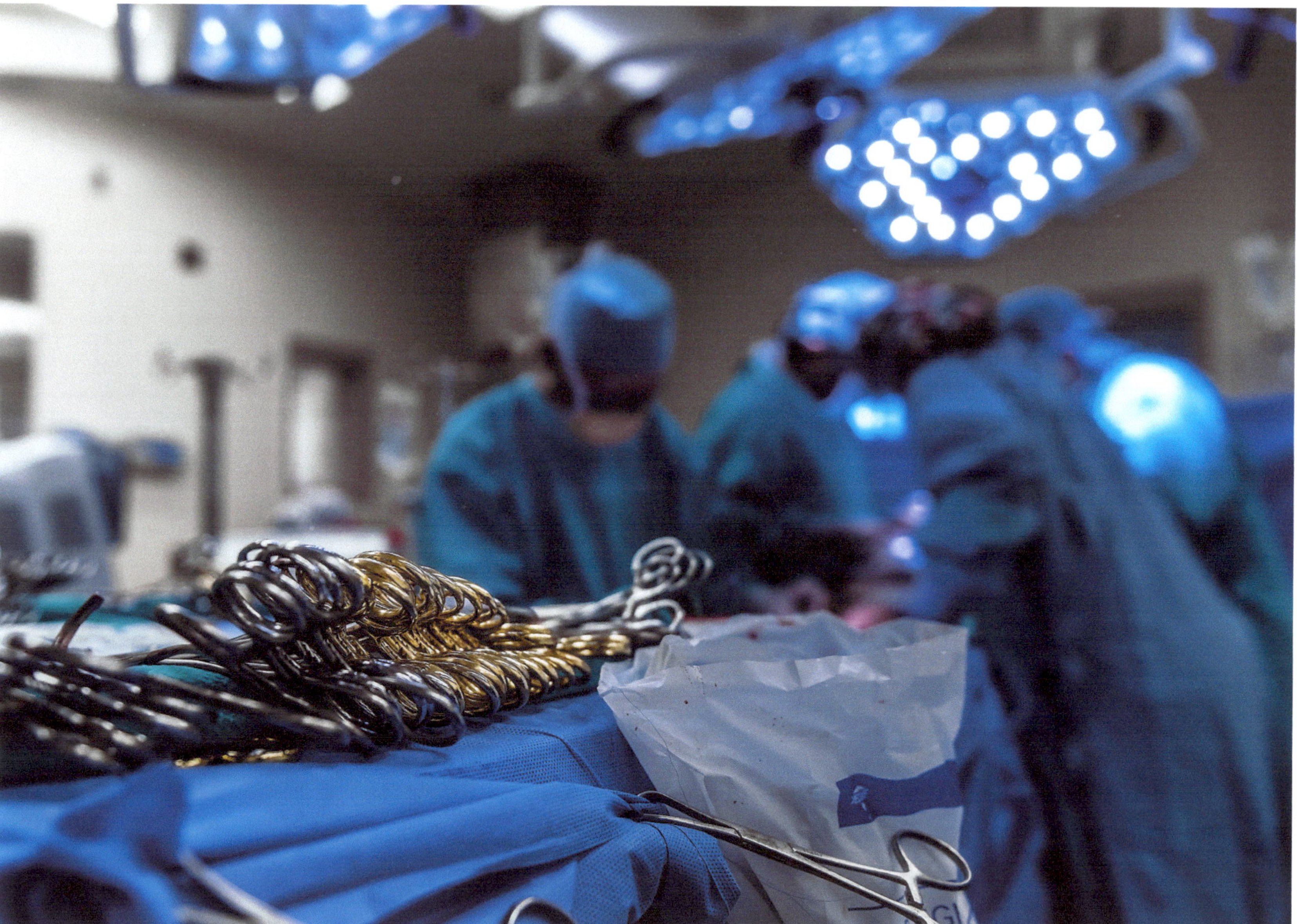

Surgery in progress

However, occasionally, the heart may awaken fibrillating, which means it is beating asynchronously. In such cases, the surgeon will de-fibrillate the heart, or jolt the heart with an electric shock, with internal electric paddles. Sometimes, the heart may be lazy or too weak, and refuse to awaken. In those cases, the surgeon will induce heart rhythm with internal pacing. The surgeon inserts pacing wires into the heart muscle, which are connected to a pacing machine. This assists the heart in beating until the heart regains its own rhythm. Pacing wires are routinely inserted on all patients, should the patient require pacing at a later stage, post-operatively.

Once the heart is beating, the anesthetist starts the ventilator, forcing the patient's lungs to breathe and mechanically begin the body's own oxygenation system. The gradual weaning from cardiopulmonary bypass begins. Typically, the CPB machine circulates blood volume at the rate of 5L per minute during the procedure. As the weaning process commences, the blood-flow rate is now reduced to 4L per minute. All observe monitors to assess patient blood pressure and heart rhythm statistics, to see how the patient's heart is able to pump blood volume on its own. After a period of time, the CPB machine is gradually reduced to 3L per minute, 2L per minute, 1L per minute, and eventually the heart is pumping its own entire blood volume. In some cases, the heart is weak and requires support to come off the CPB machine. In those cases, the anesthetist will administer pharmacologic drugs intravenously, to assist the heart in coming off pump. Typically, these aids are drugs such as dopamine, dobutamine, epinephrine, and norepinephrine. They work in various ways to elevate blood pressure, by vasoconstriction, which constricts blood vessels, or by increasing contractility of the heart muscle. This patient's heart came off pump without any pharmacologic support.

Once the patient is weaned off the CPB machine, the patient's rehabilitated heart is now functioning independently. At this point, the surgeon first disconnects the venous cannula from the patient followed by the aortic cannula. Patient is now off all mechanical support, and the heart and lungs are functioning, unassisted.

The next phase is to reverse the anti-coagulation process of the blood initiated prior to going on cardiopulmonary bypass to prevent blood from clotting within the machine. The anesthetist begins reversing the heparin-induced blood thinning, by intravenously administering a drug called protamine so that blood can resume its normal clotting function.

Once normal blood clotting is established, which can sometimes take a while, and there is insignificant oozing in the chest, the surgeon begins with chest closure. He first inserts three chest tubes through the skin into the chest, two overlying the heart and one in the left lung cavity, to allow for drainage of any blood collecting in the chest cavity after the chest is closed, post operatively. The pacemaker wires are also brought through the skin. The chest is closed using eight sternal wires, which the surgeon inserts through the bone to bind the sternum together. The first assistant has closed the incision on the leg used for harvesting the vein grafts. The procedure was a success and is now complete. Surgeons have left the operating room after almost five hours of intense concentration.

In my mind, catharsis of watching the patient come off pump was palpable.

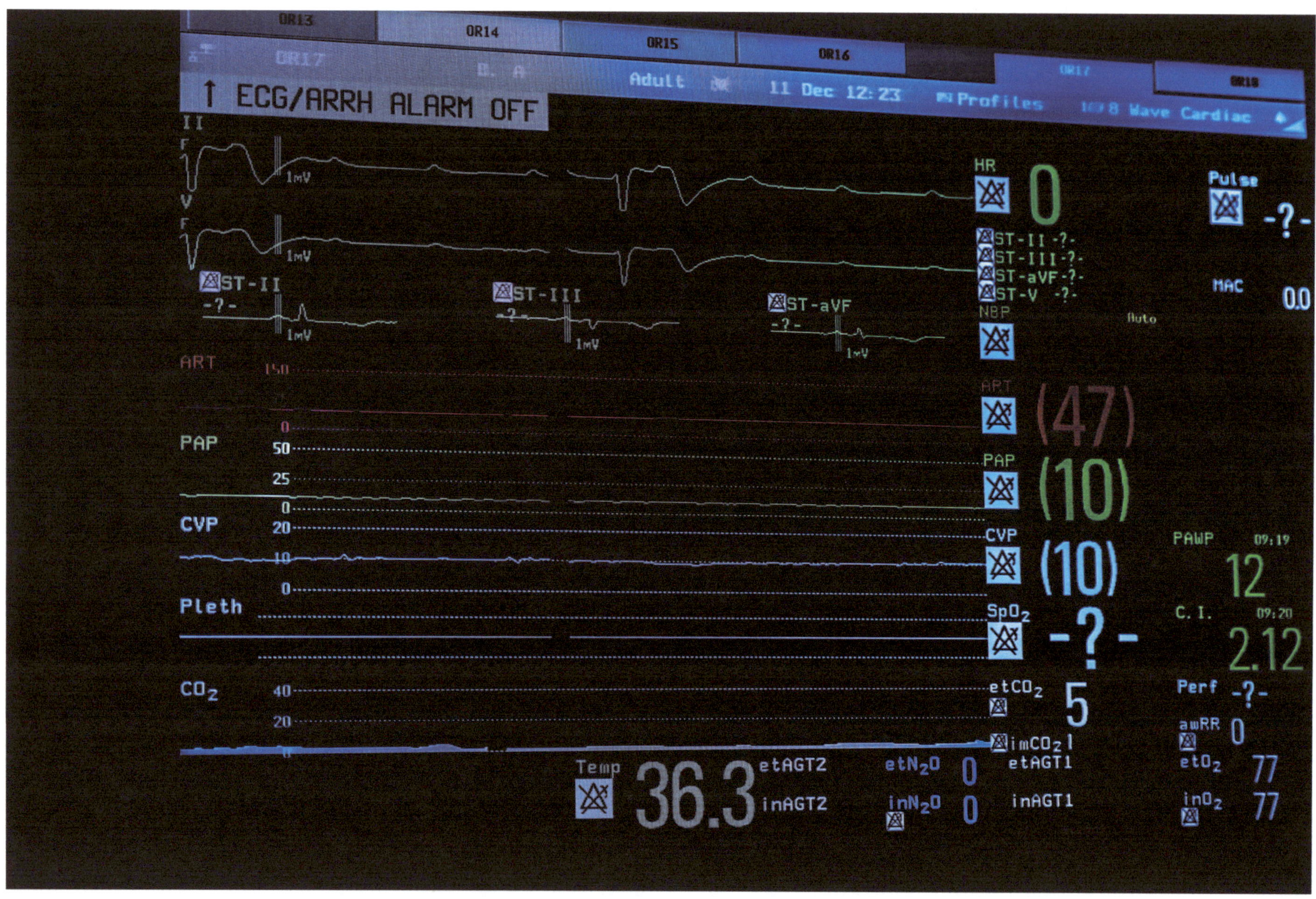

Hot shot has been administered and the aortic cross clamp removed—within minutes rudiments of a heart rhythm erupt

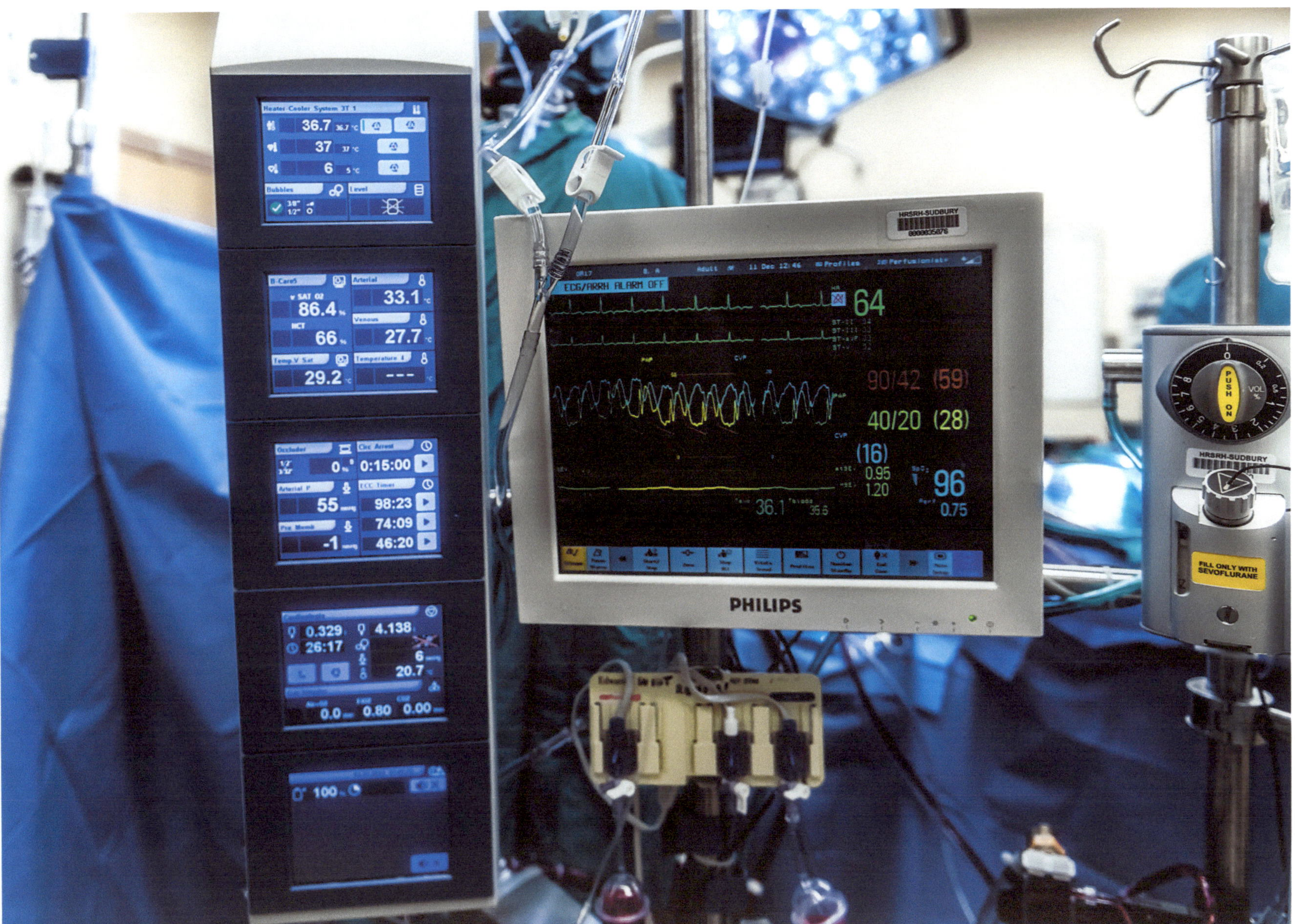

ECG monitor indicating the heart has now resumed a sinus rhythm at 64 beat per minute

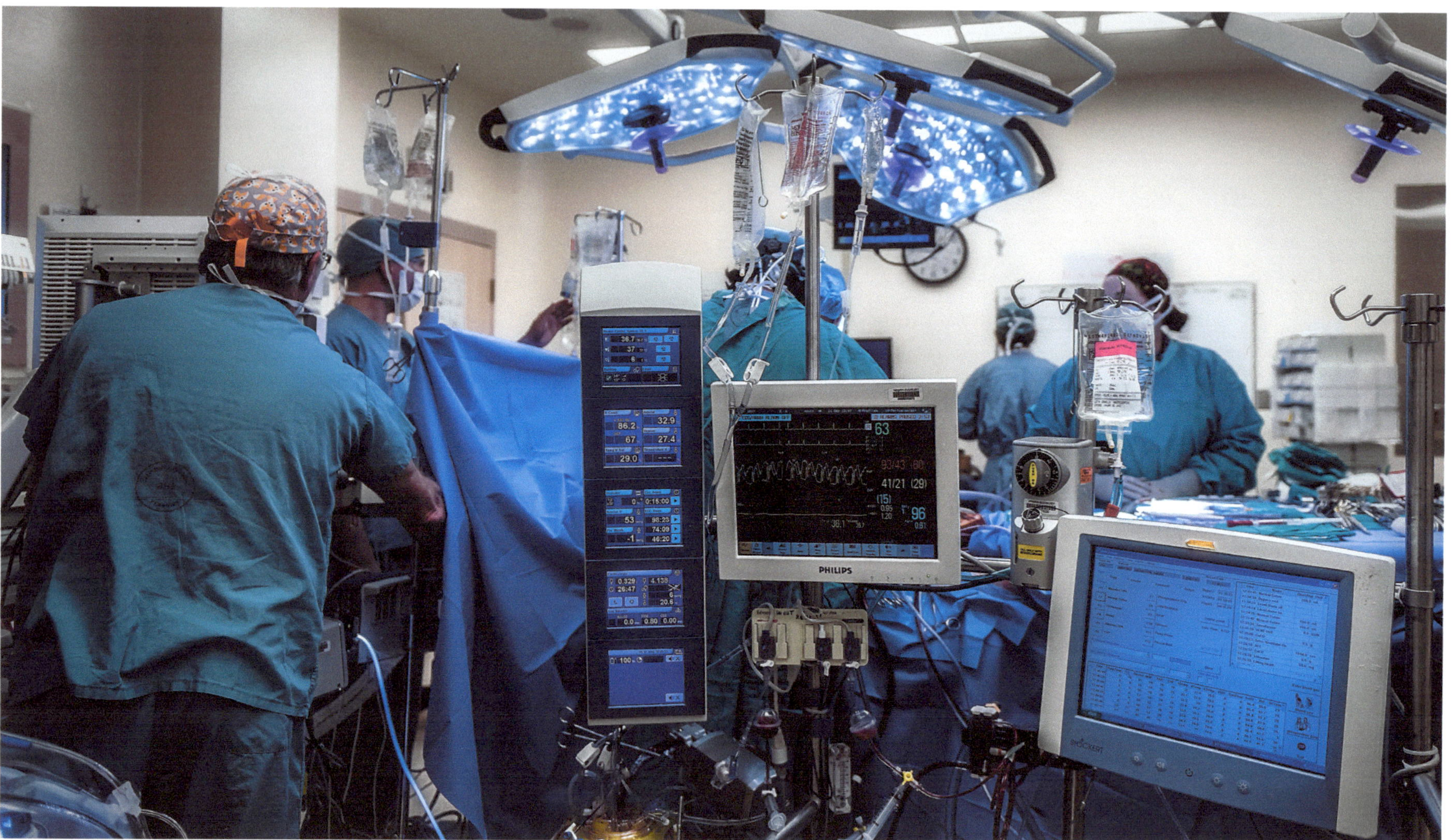

Perfusionist monitoring patient statistics

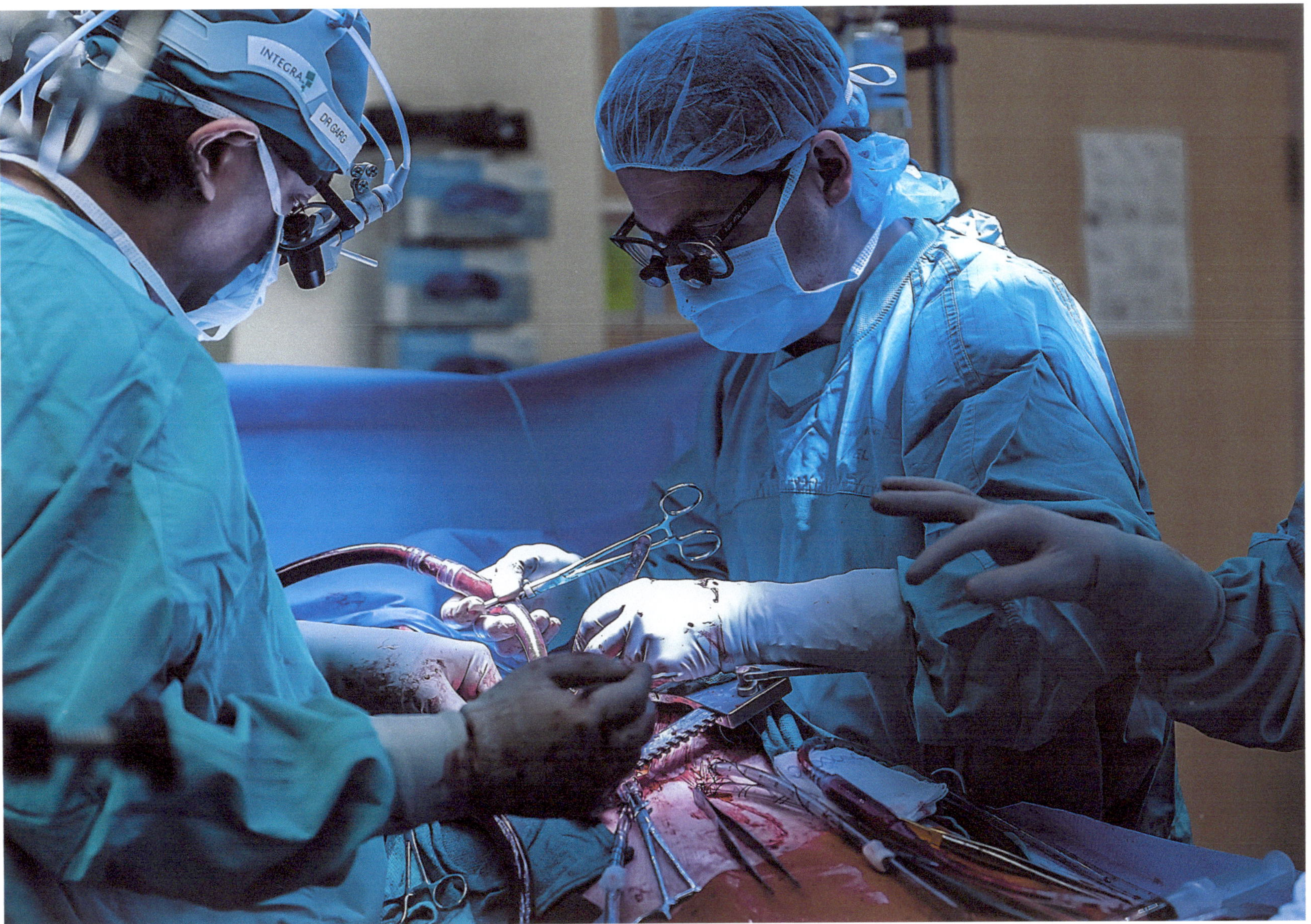

The patient is successfully weaned from the CPB machine, the venous cannula connected to the machine is being removed, followed by the aortic cannula

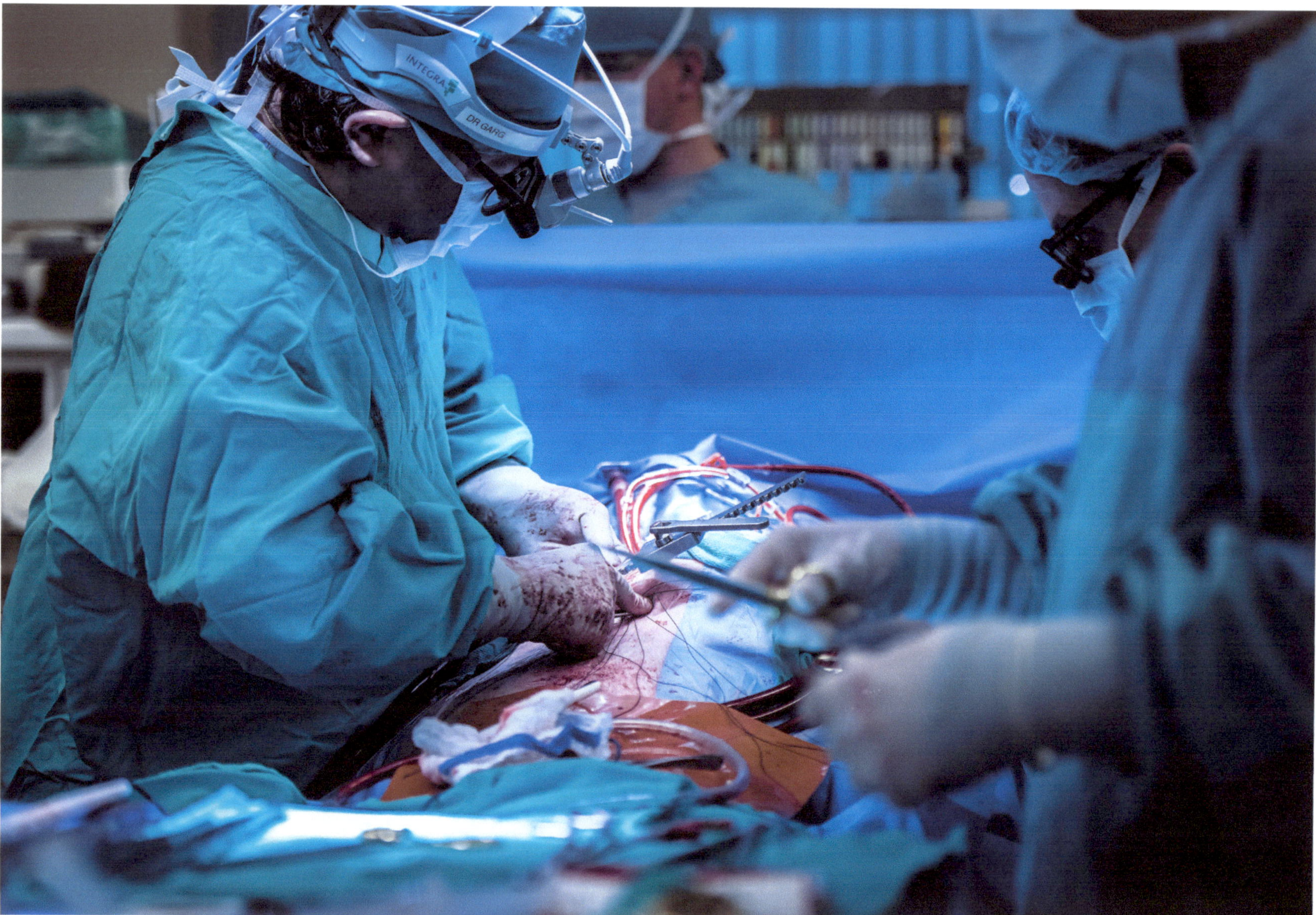

Surgeon piercing the skin for chest tube insertion

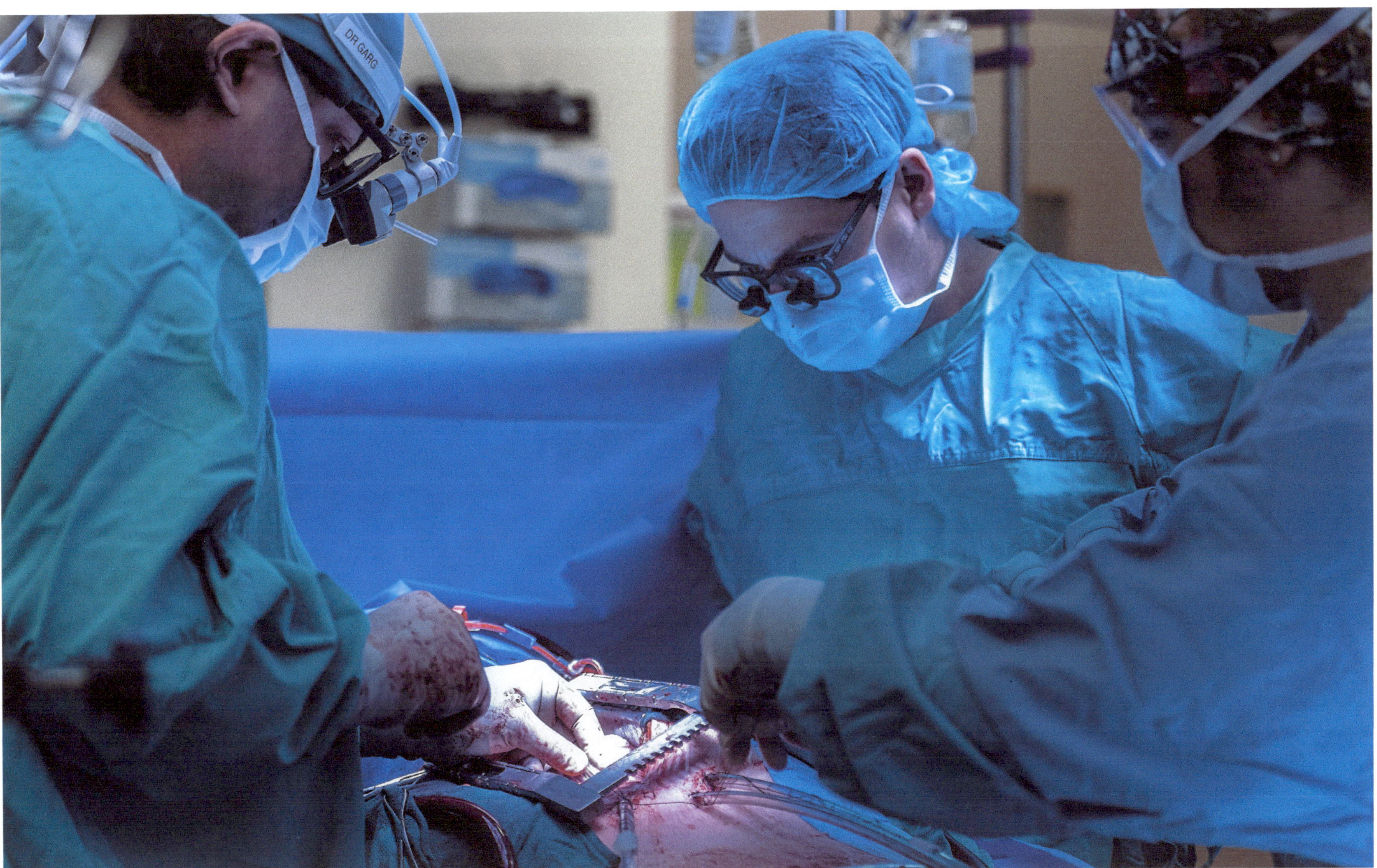

Chest tubes being positioned over the heart

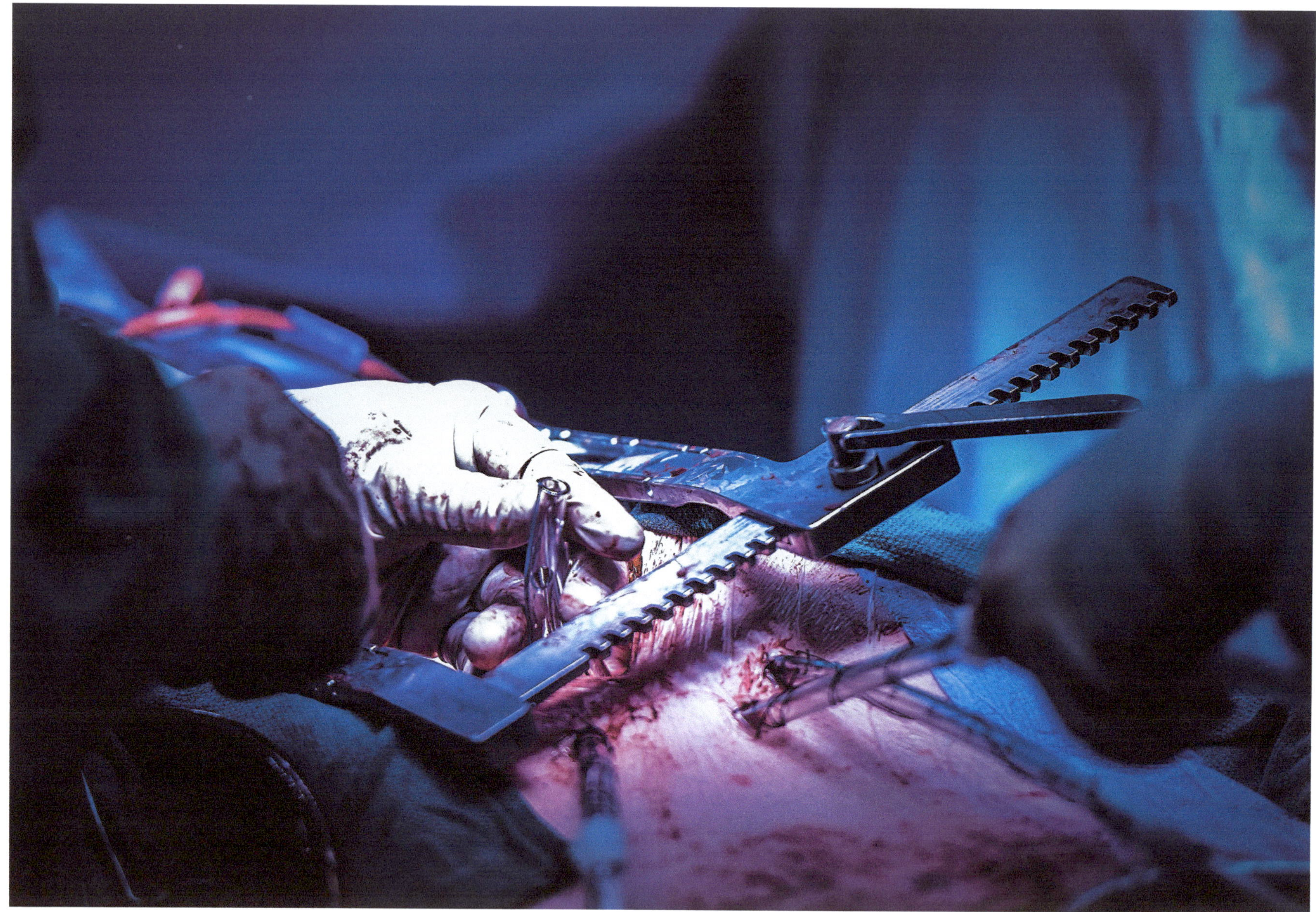

Chest tubes secured in place with sutures; two chest tubes overlying the heart, and one within the left chest cavity

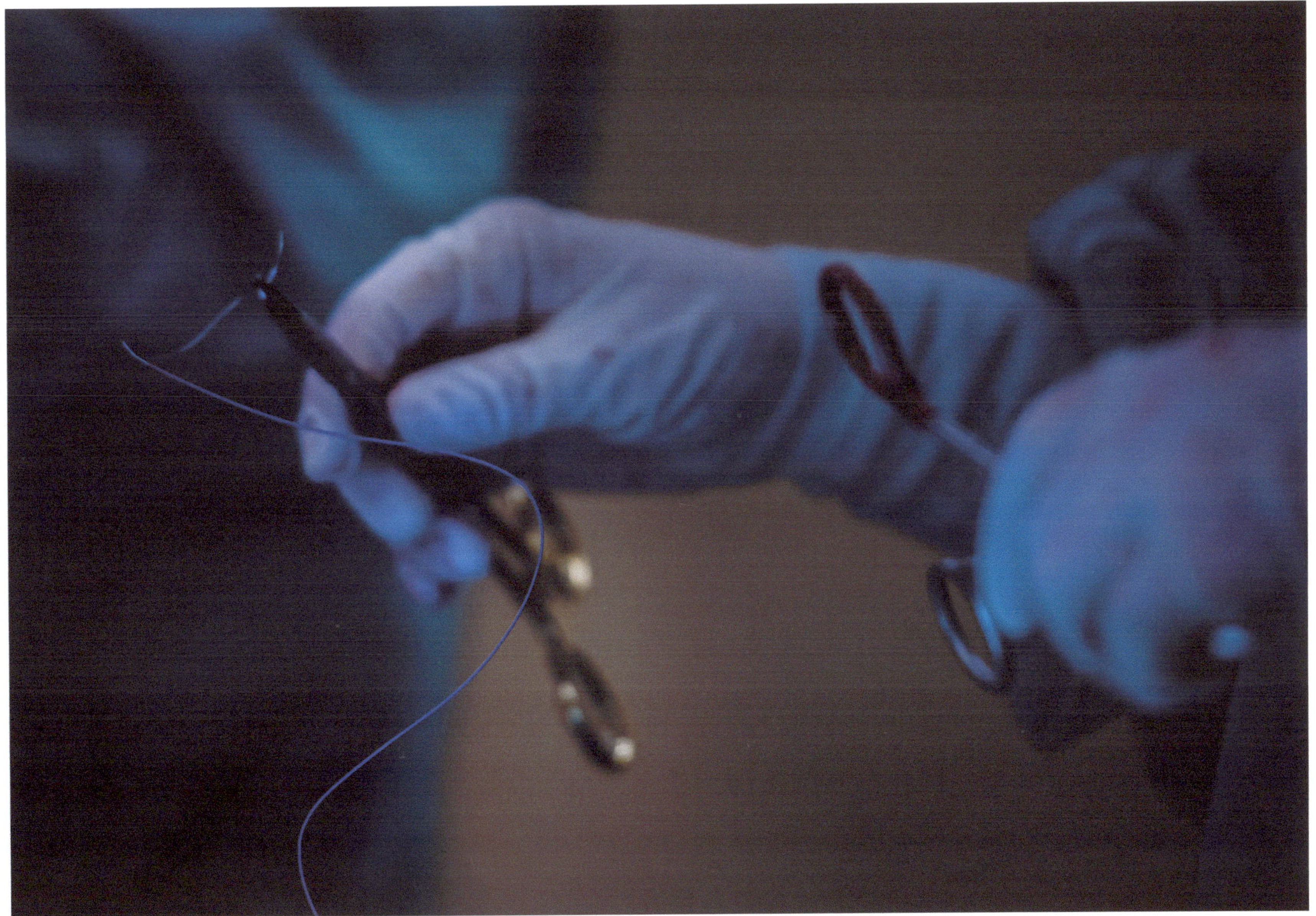

Nurse hands the pacemaker wire for insertion. The surgeon will insert the wire by bringing the curved needle through the heart muscle.

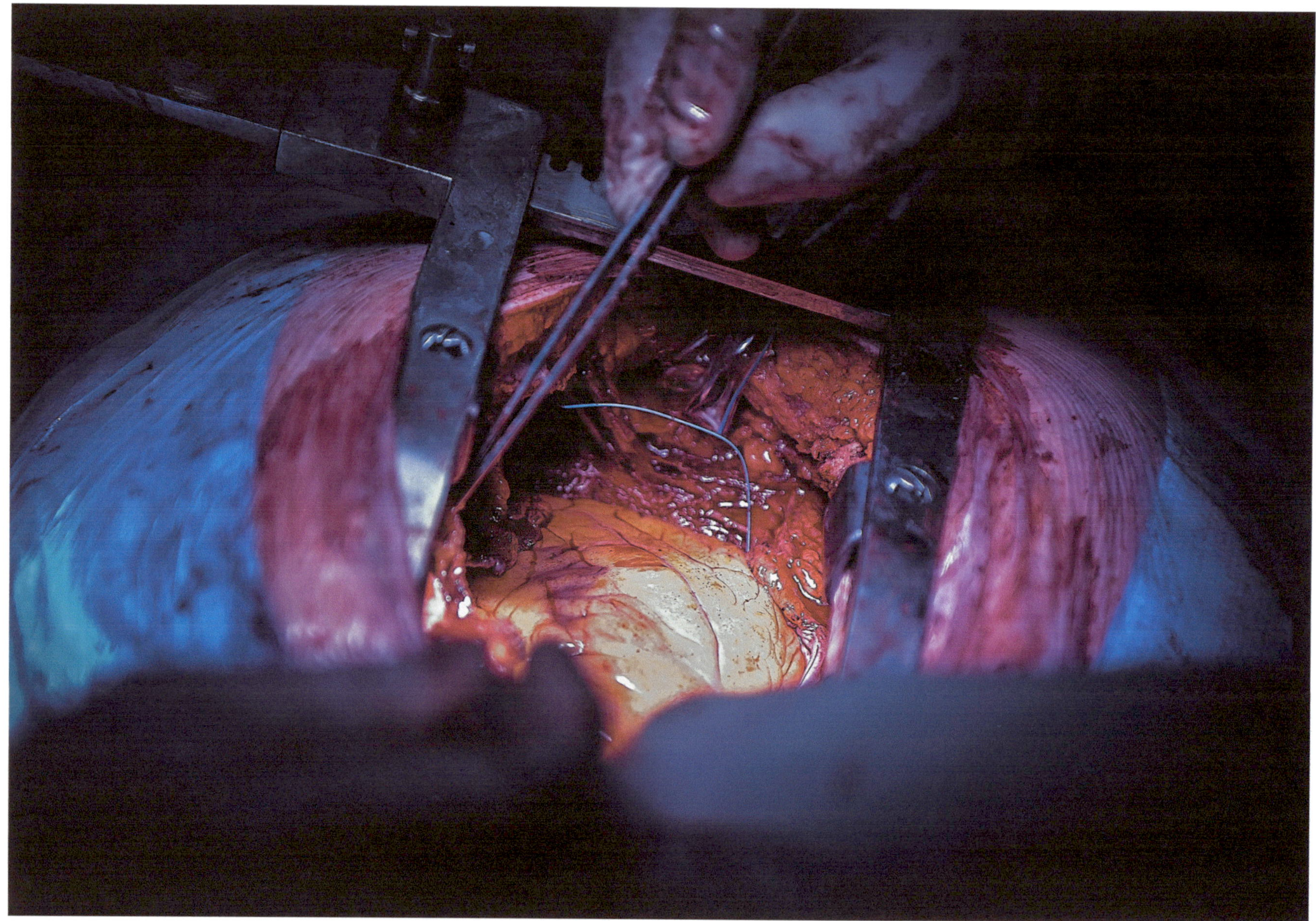

Blue pacemaker wire lodged in position at the bottom of the heart

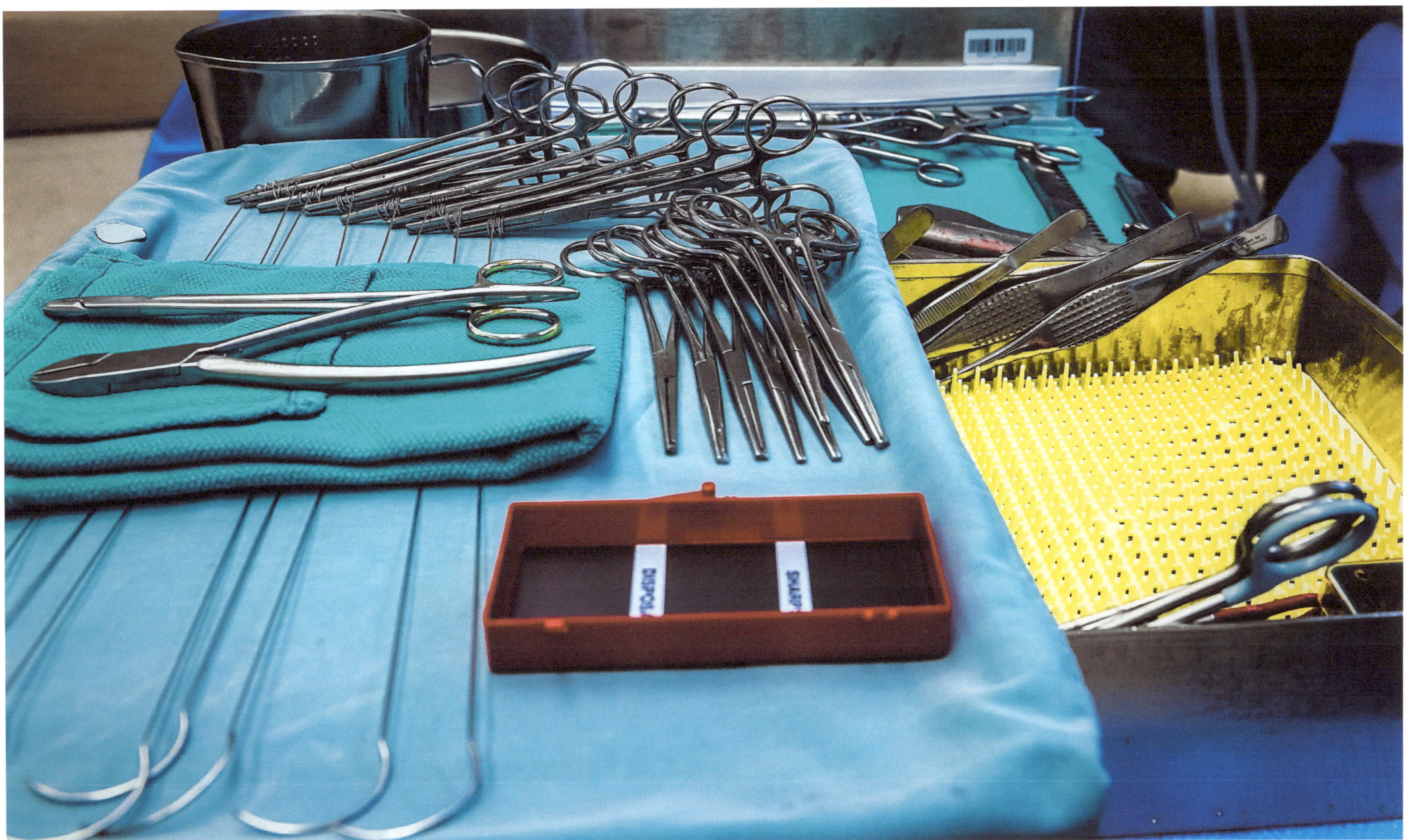

Sternal wires used for chest closure

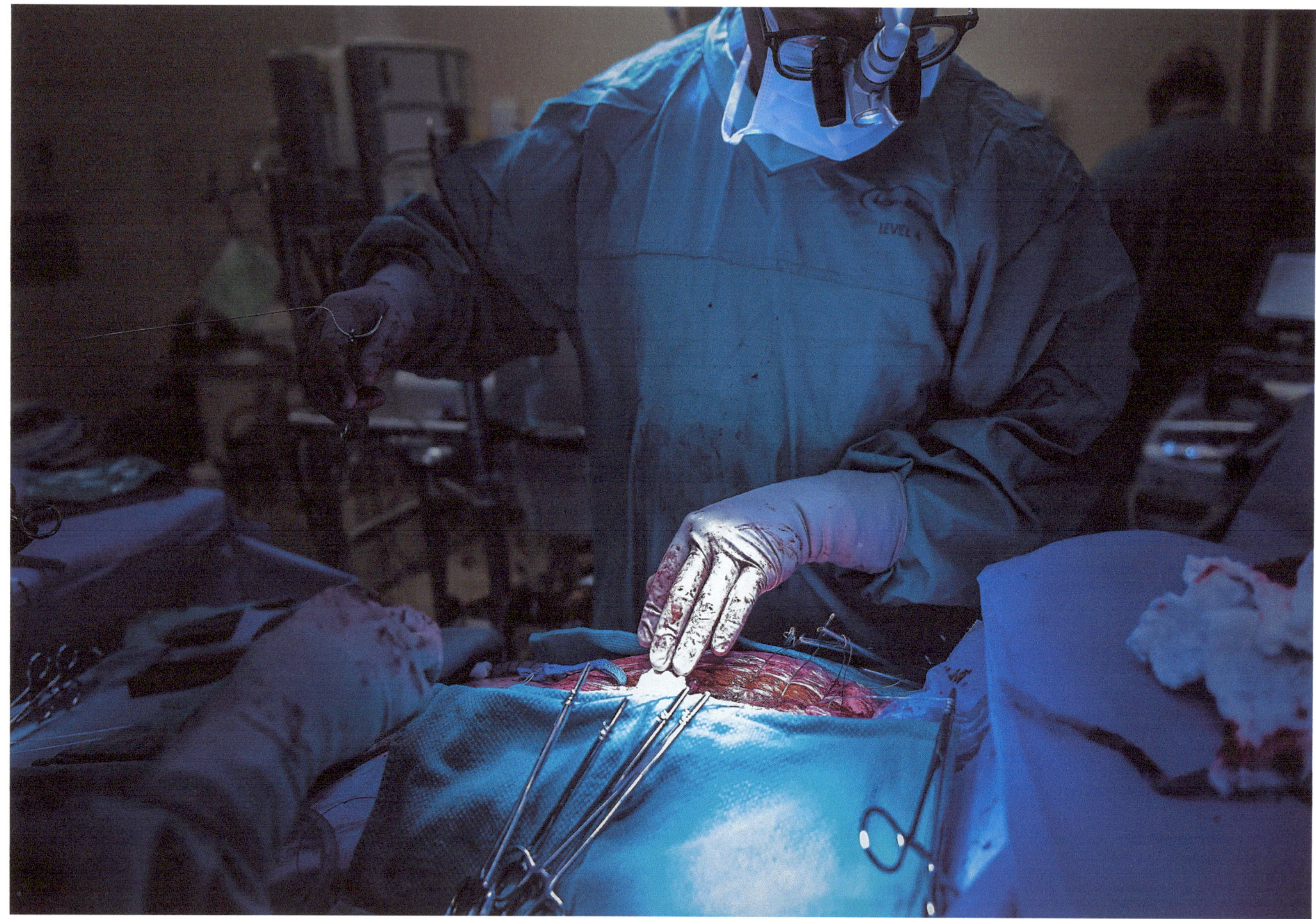

Sternal wires inserted along either side of sternum

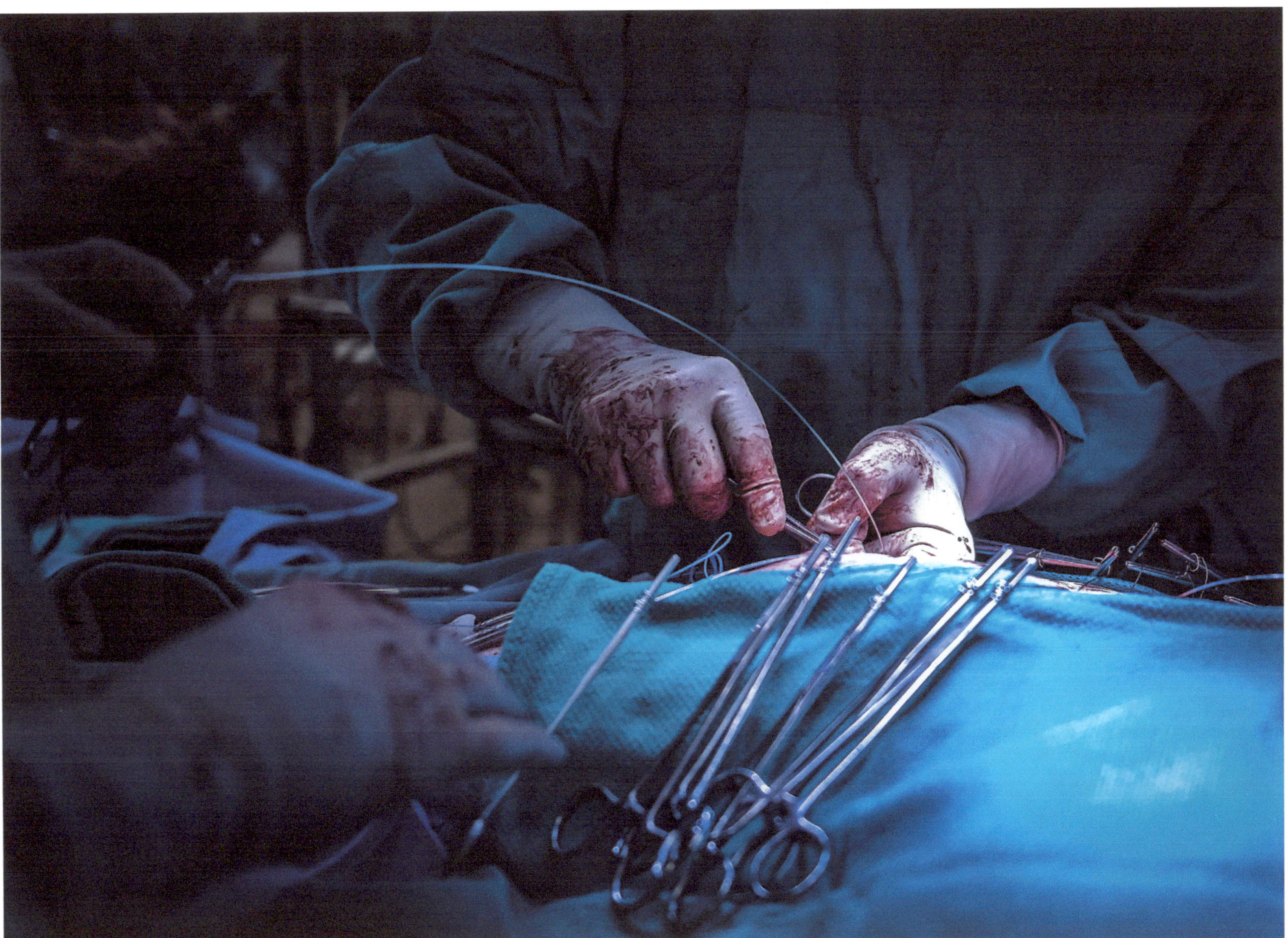

Sternal wires clasped in place with Kocher clamps

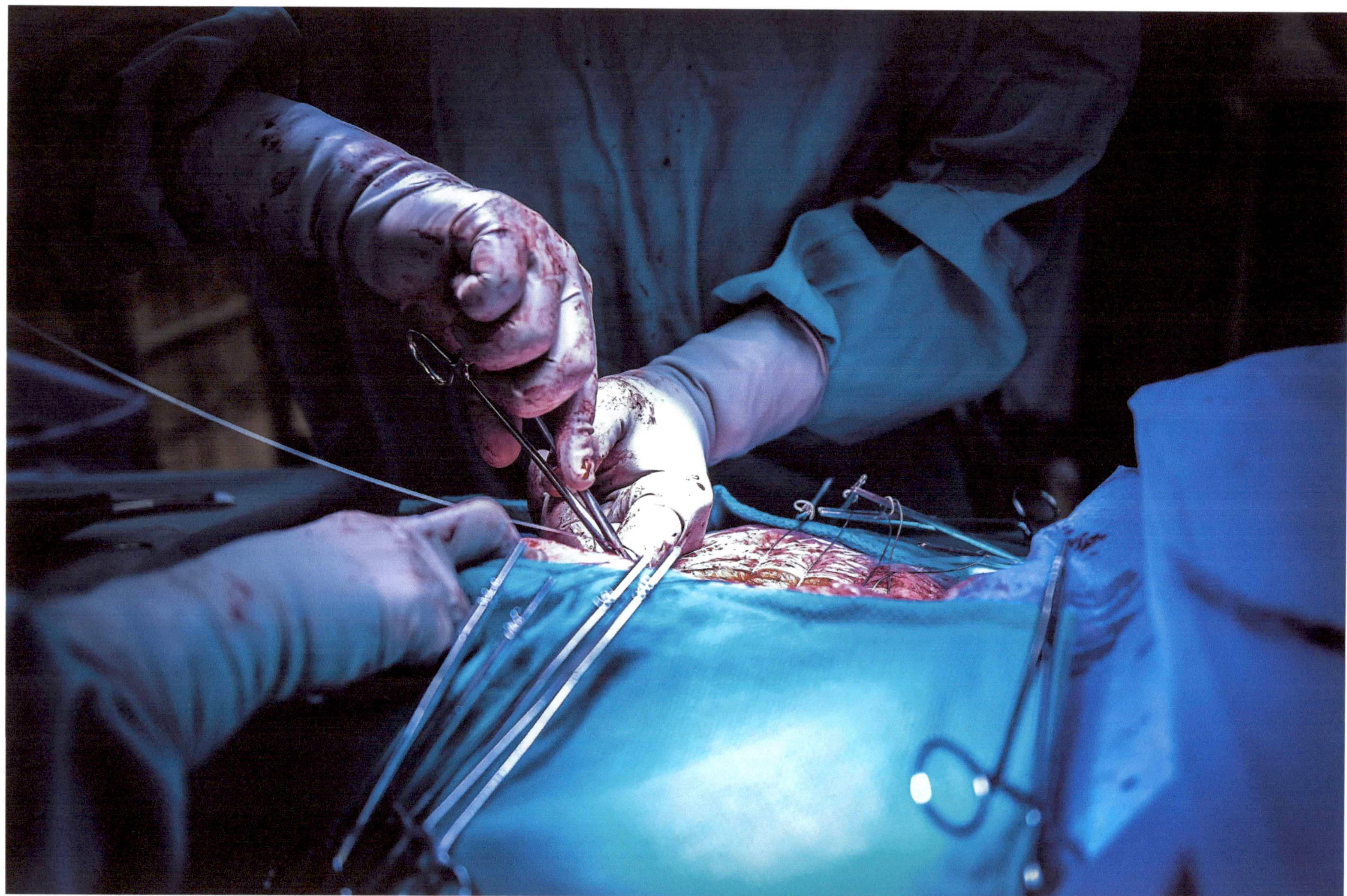

Closure process—assistant holds one end of the wire while surgeon inserts the other end

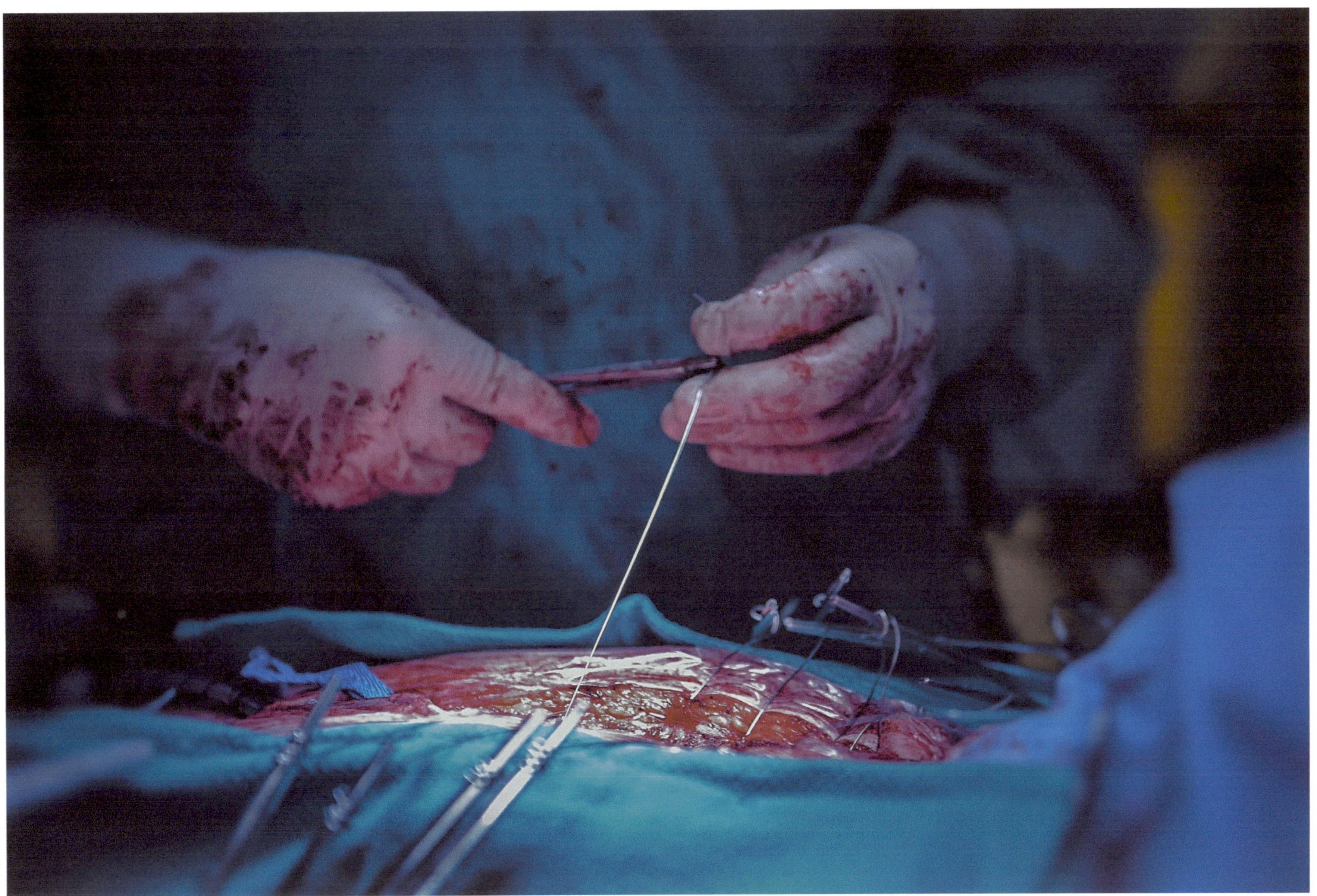

Sternal wires are brought together to bind the sternum together

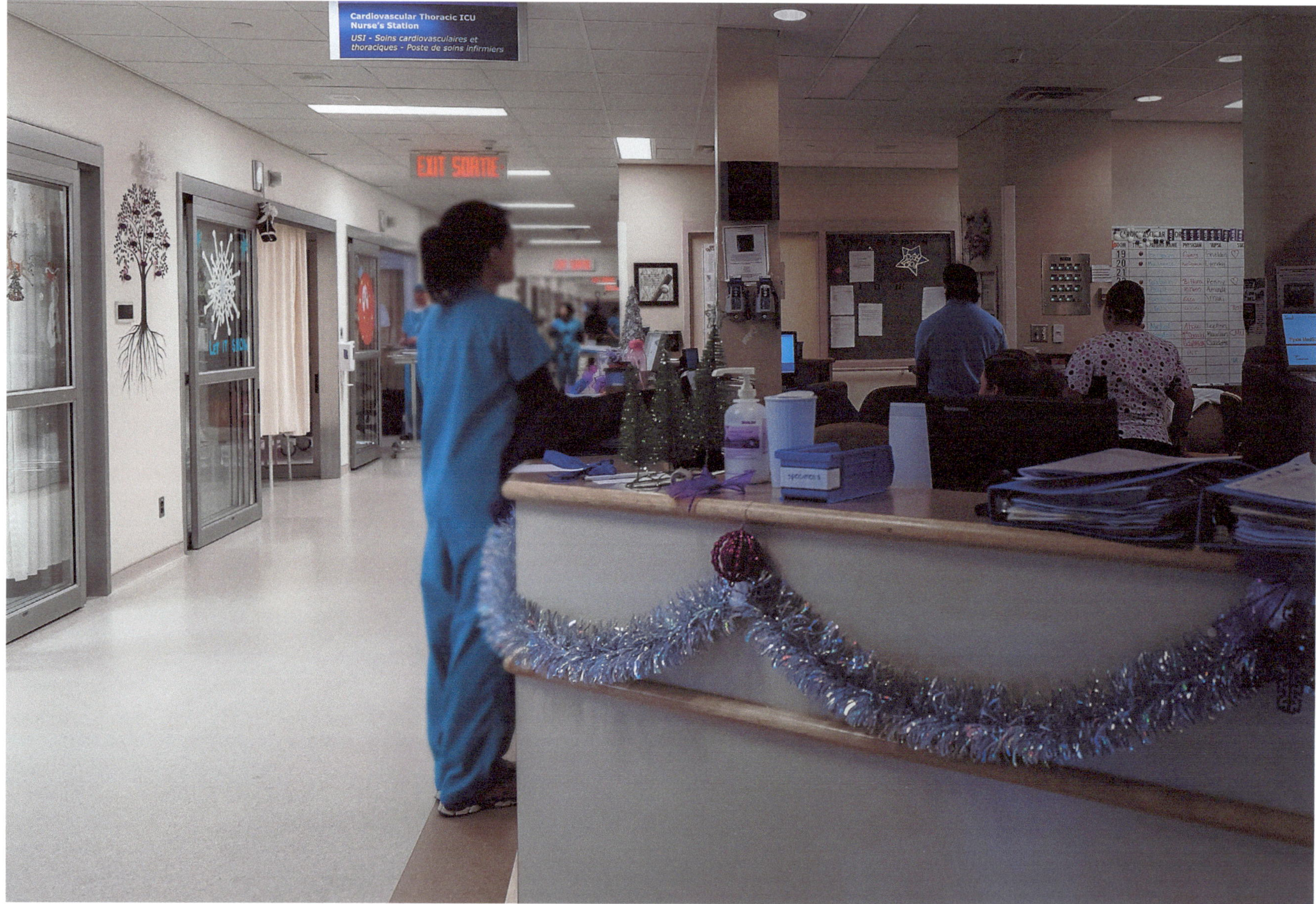

Intensive Care Unit

Intensive Care

At this point, the operating room nurses take over, and the anesthetist remains at the patient's side, monitoring patient vital signs.

Nurses bandage the chest and leg wounds. The patient is then wrapped tightly in a sheet placed beneath the patient before surgery. An underlying pad is lifted by nurses and staff to carefully transfer the patient onto the Intensive Care Unit (ICU) bed.

Patient is on a warming blanket, and portable monitors are moved with the patient. The anesthetist, perfusionist, and nurses wheel the patient to the ICU.

Here, the next several hours are critical. Intensivists in the ICU take over care and carefully monitor the patient's vital statistics as the patient begins the recovery process of waking up from anesthesia. Typically, chest tubes inserted during surgery are removed two days after surgery, and the pacemaker wire is removed prior to discharge.

Remarkably, this patient was awake a few hours after surgery and was sitting in bed twelve hours later. He was discharged from hospital in five days. Seen in a three-month follow-up visit at Dr. Garg's office, the patient was doing extremely well, grateful for a new lease on life.

The following photographs describe this phase.

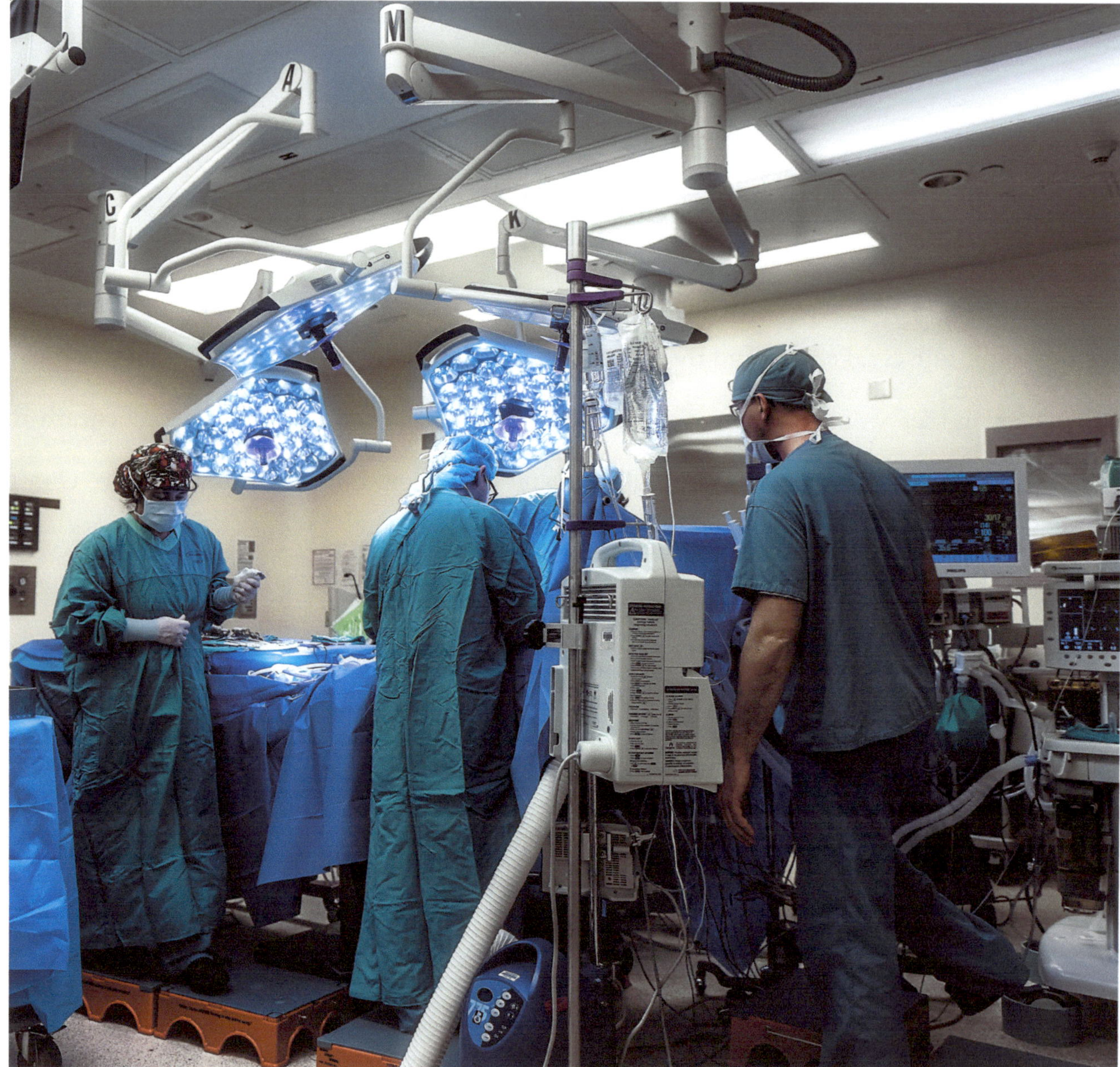

Procedure is complete

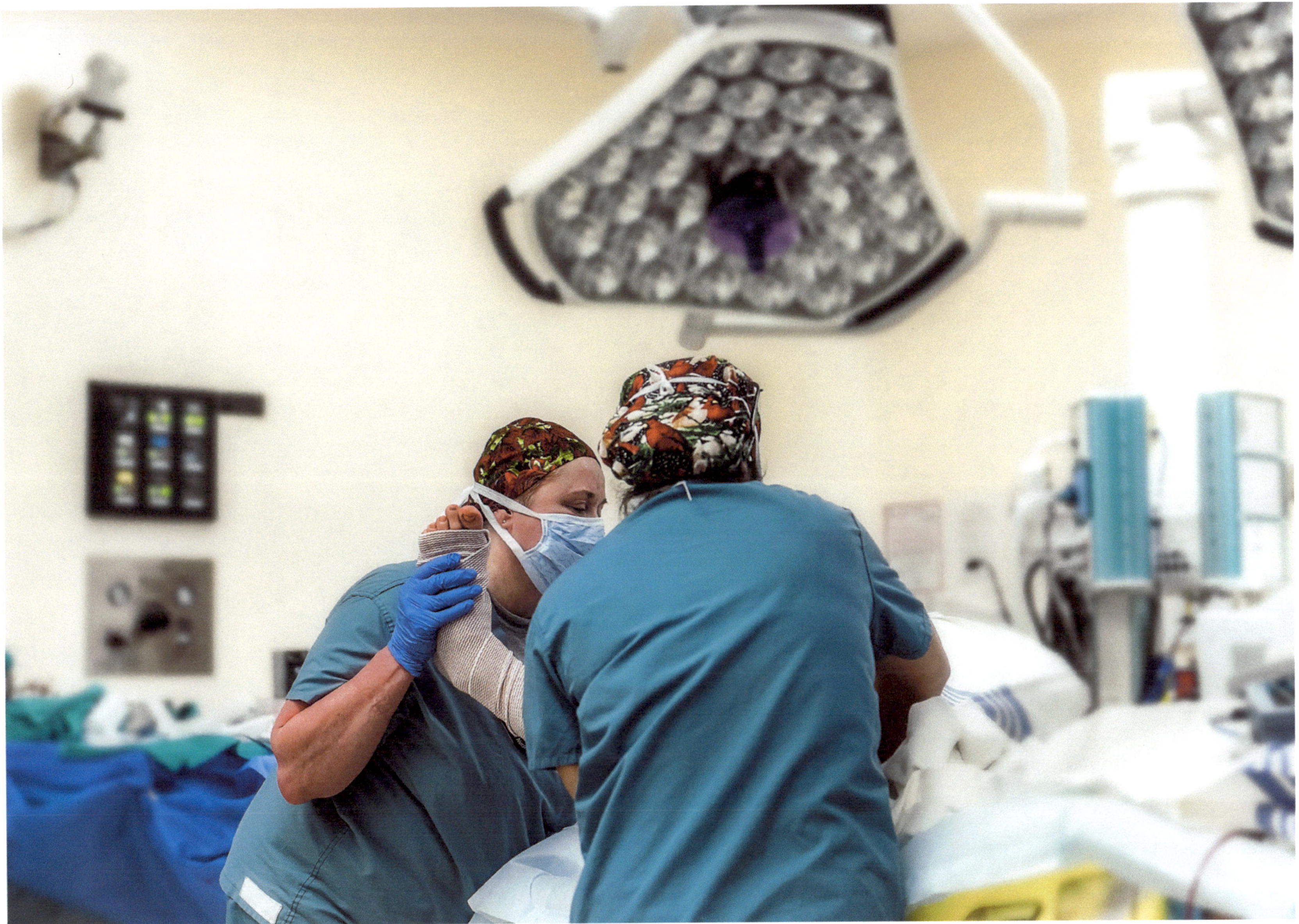

Nurses apply a compressive binding to the leg incision

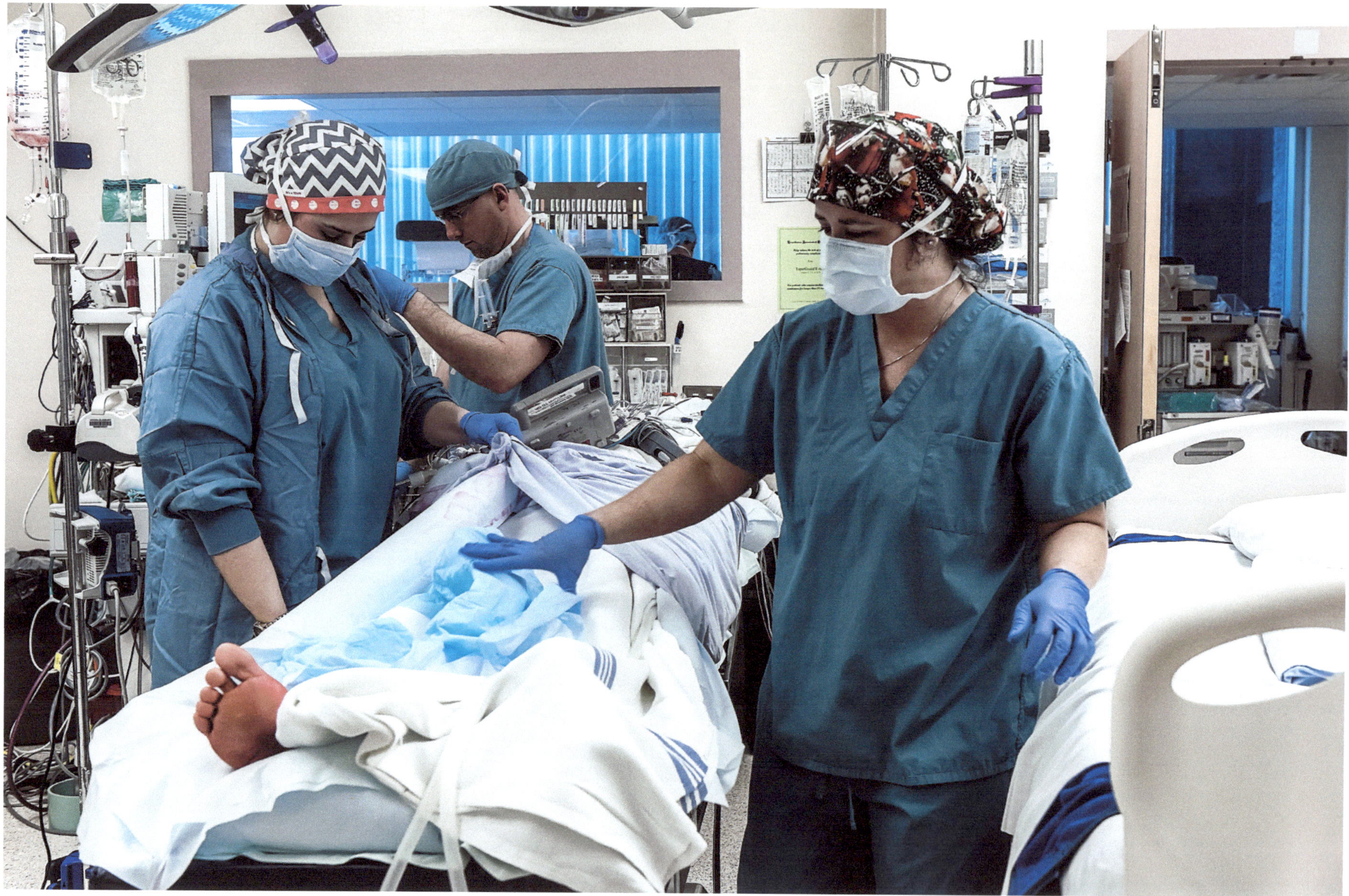

Patient wrapped in a warming blanket is ready for transfer to the ICU bed

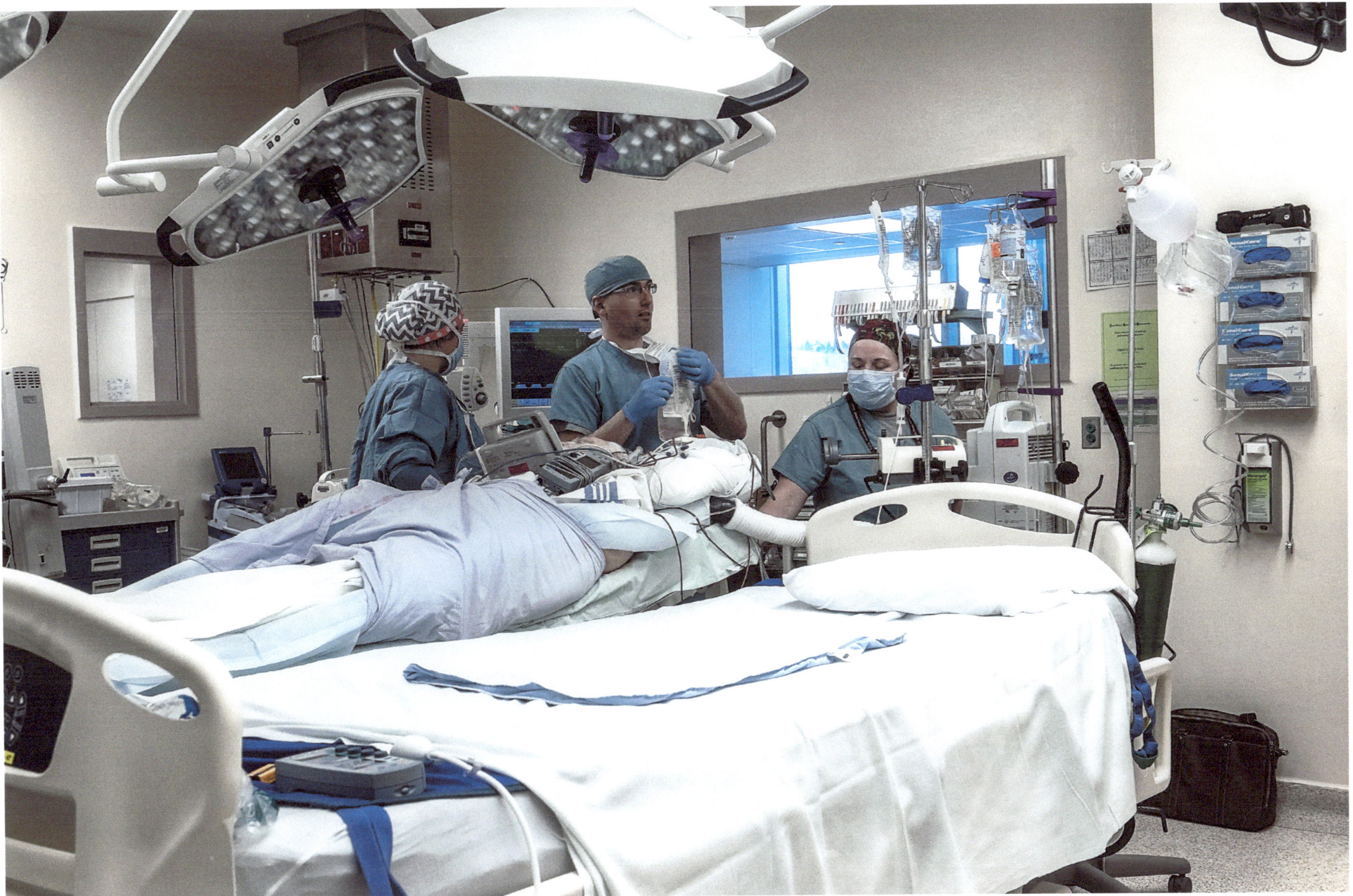

ICU bed is brought in and placed alongside the patient on the operating room table

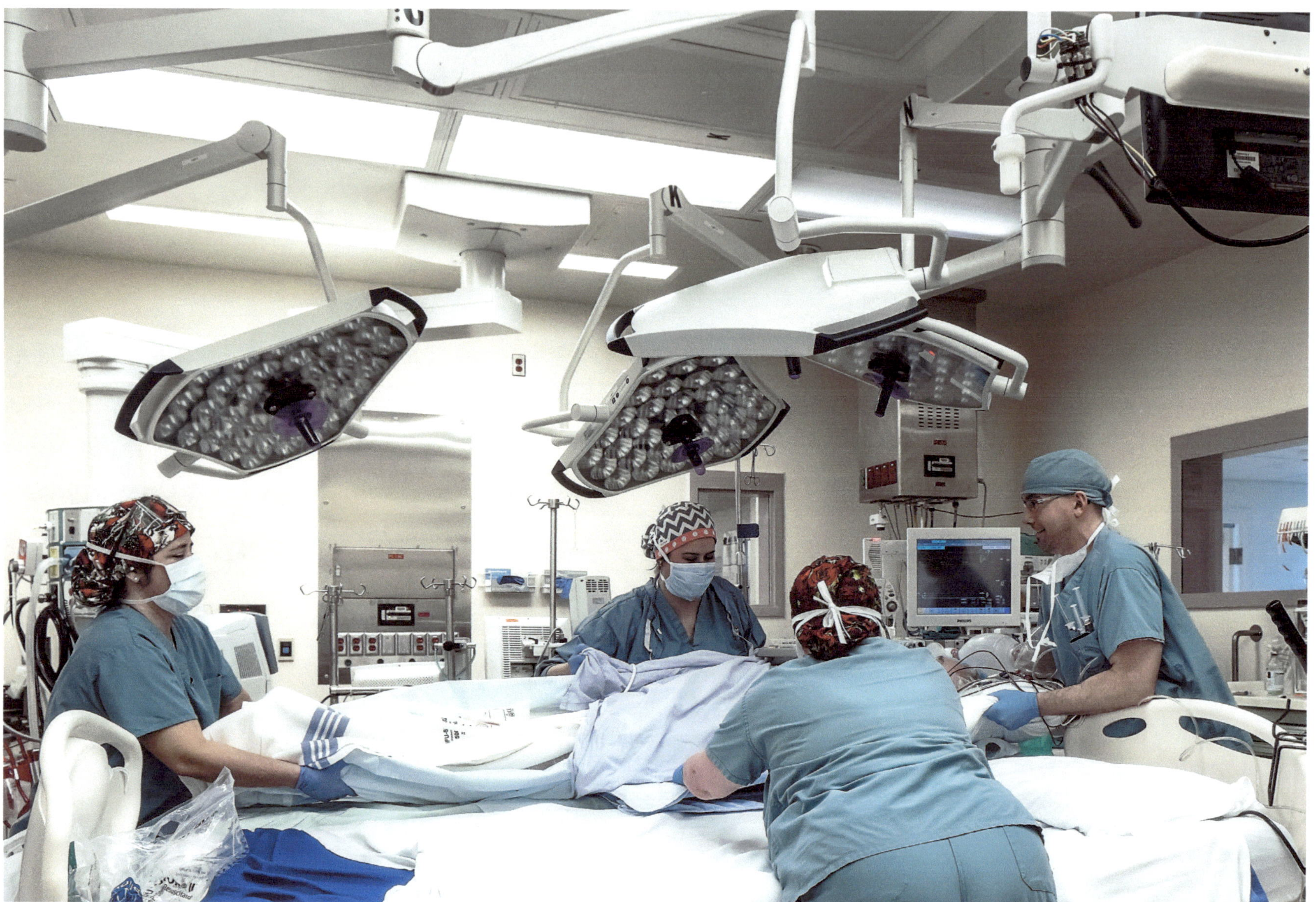

Nurses and anesthetist simultaneously grasp the sheets and pad beneath the patient

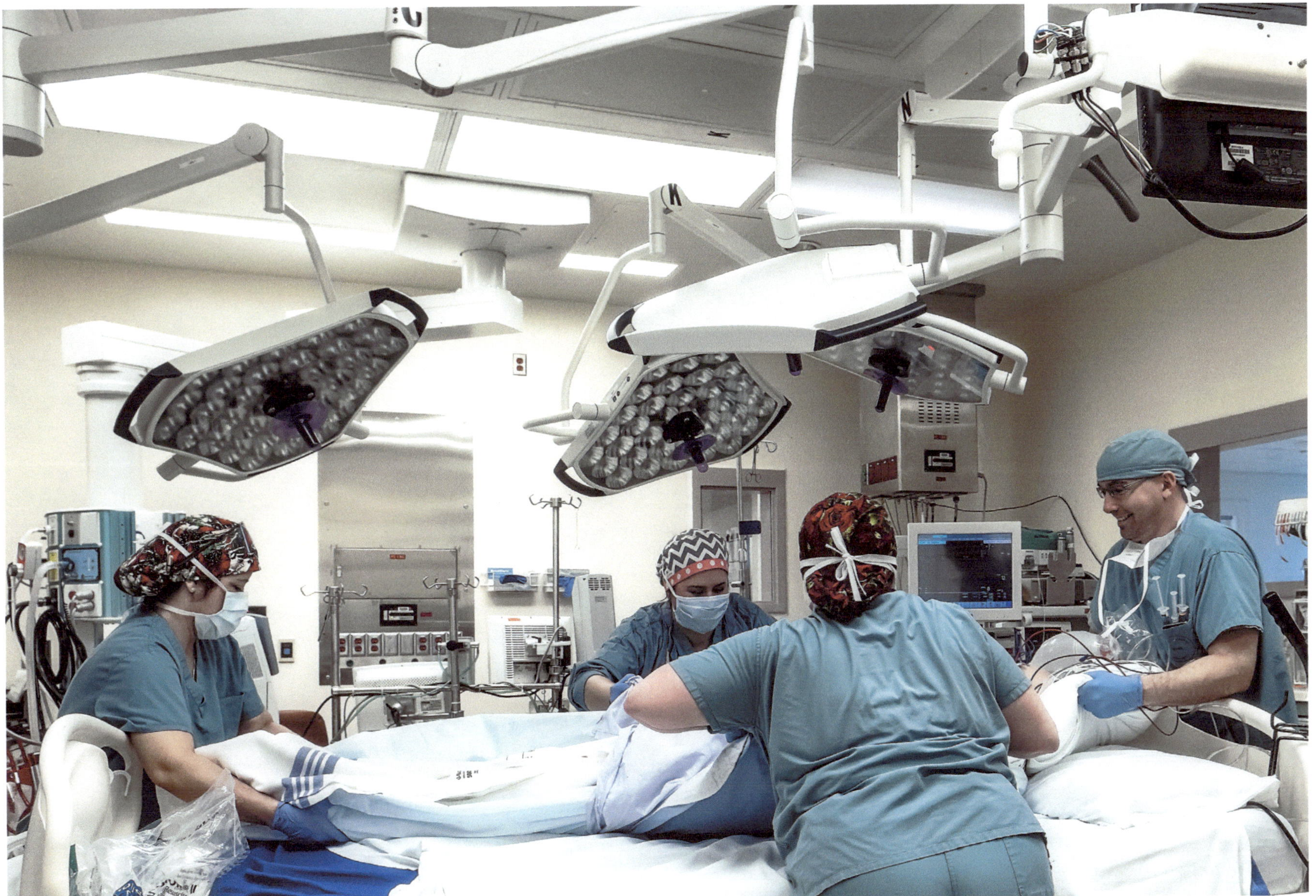

Then, carefully timing the shift, they slide the patient onto the ICU bed by pulling the sheets, pad and pillow simultaneously—a team effort

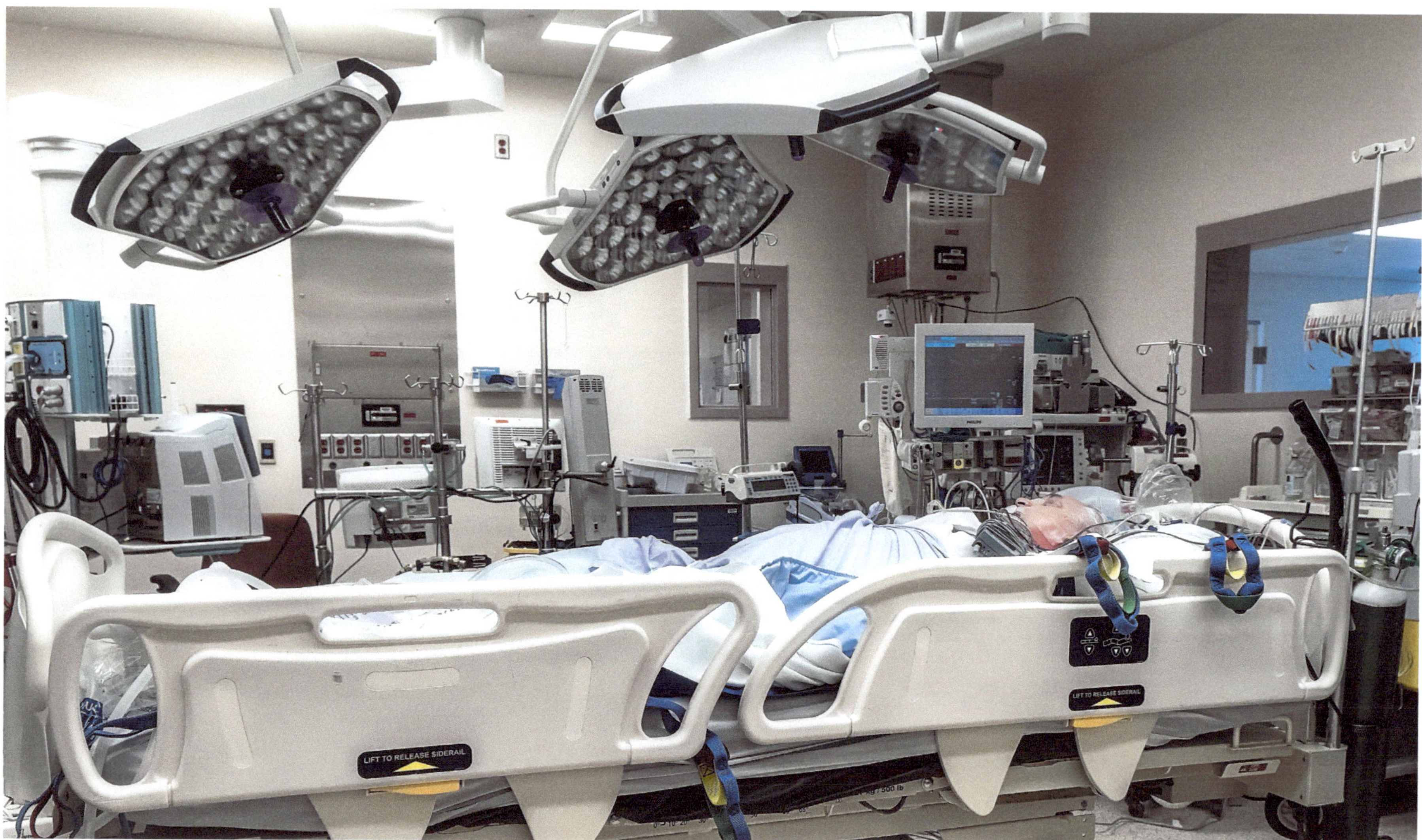

Patient is secure on the ICU bed

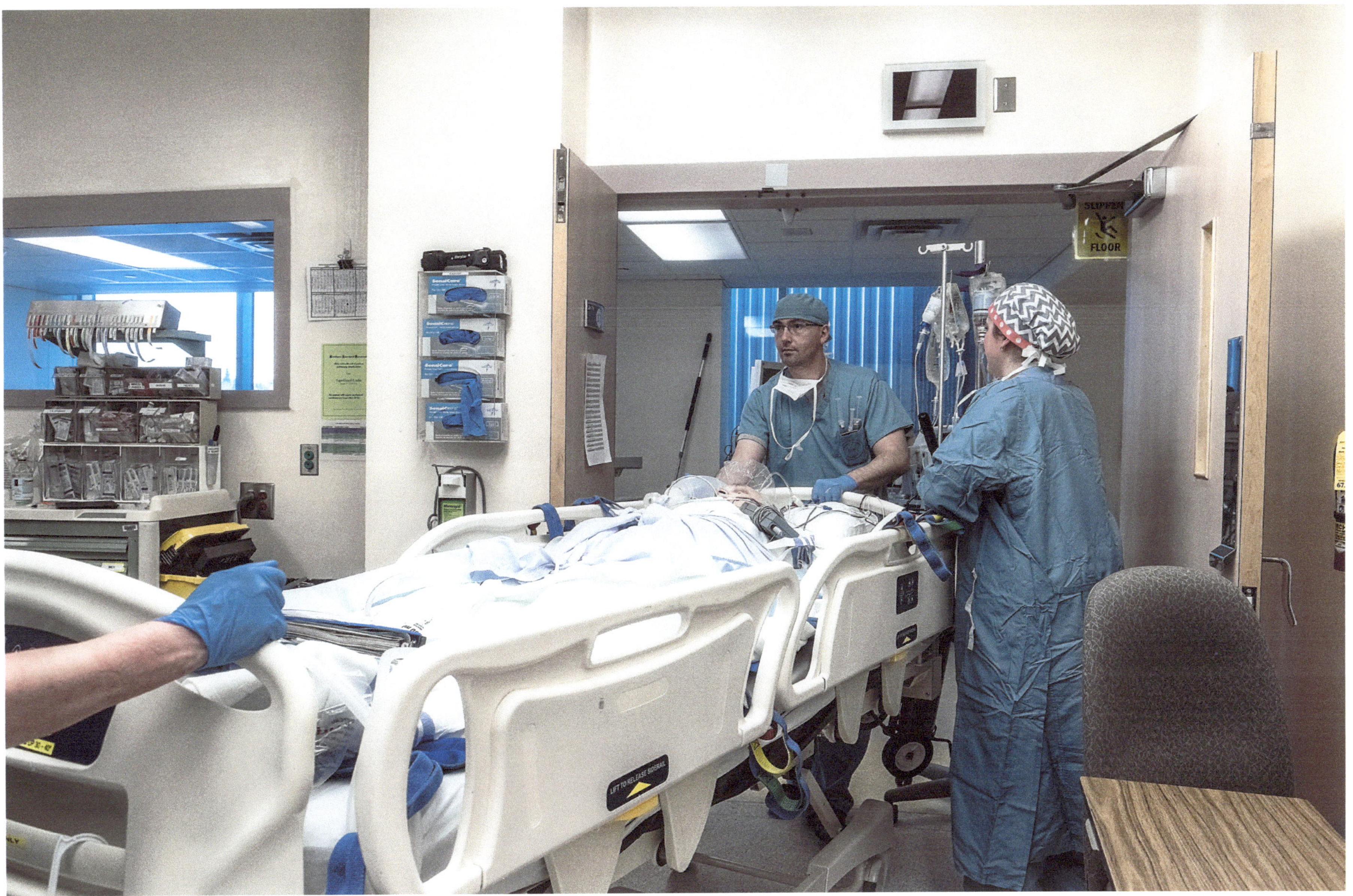

Patient is rolled out of the operating theatre, anesthetist is alongside

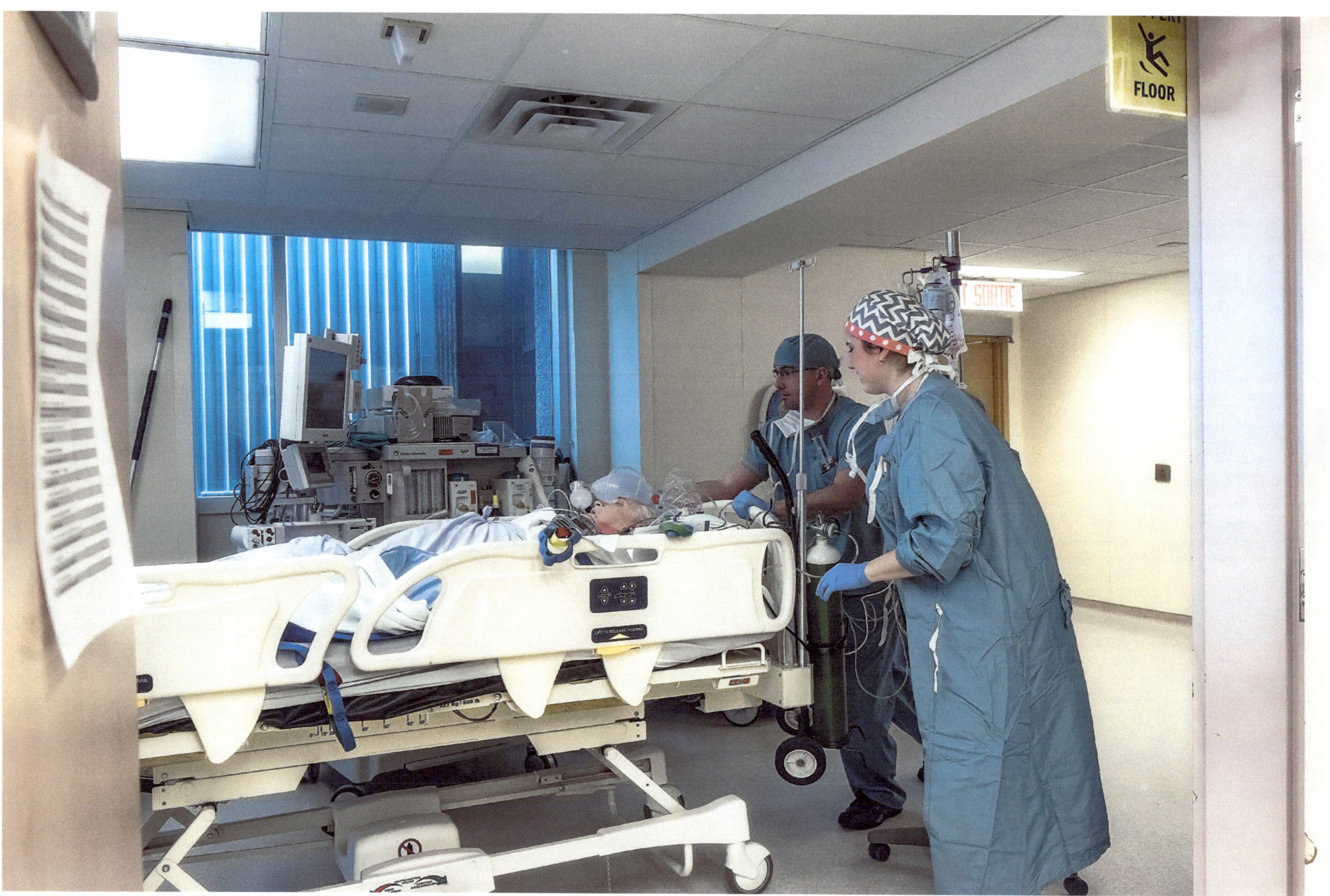

Out of Operating Room 17

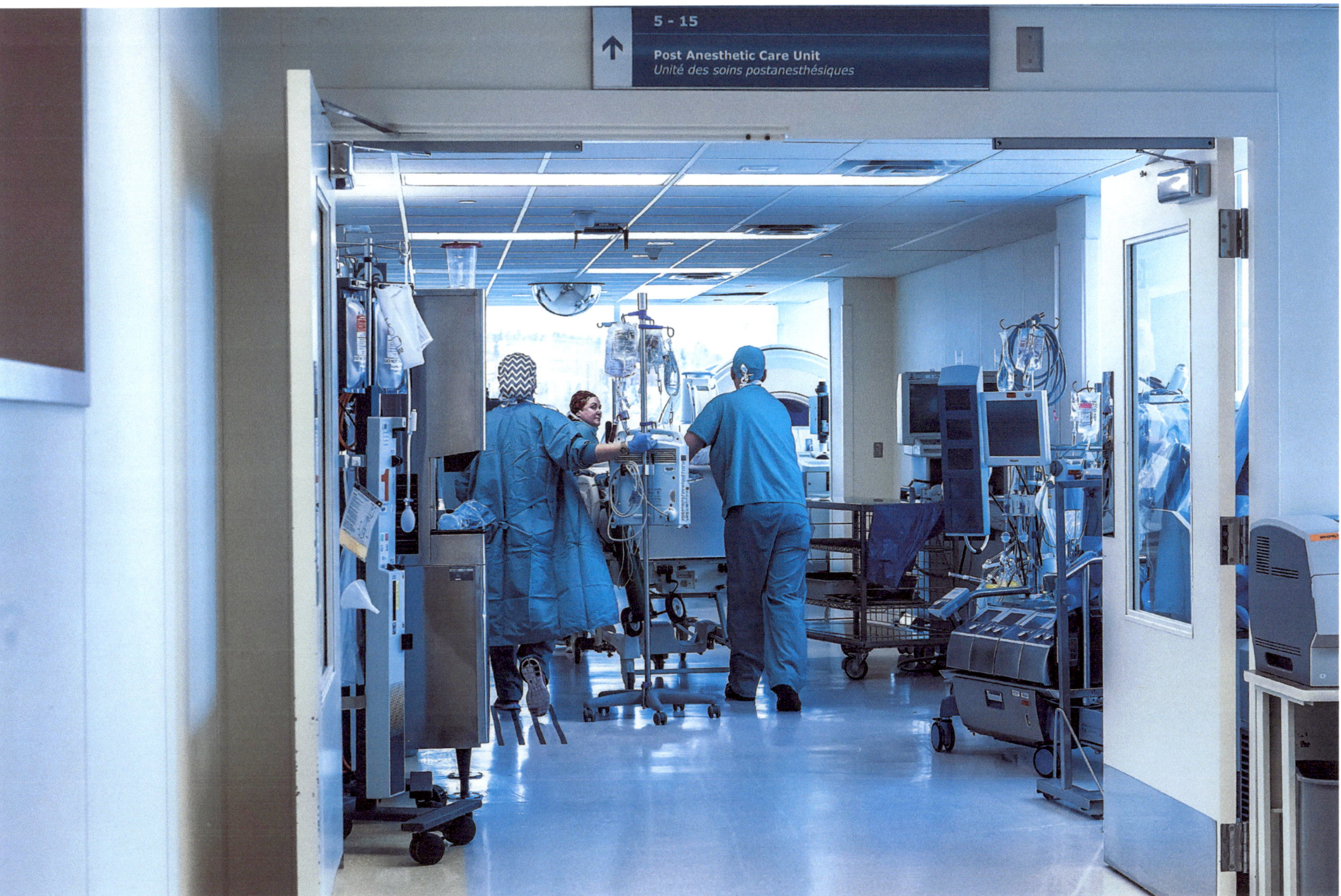

Patient is en route to the Intensive Care Unit

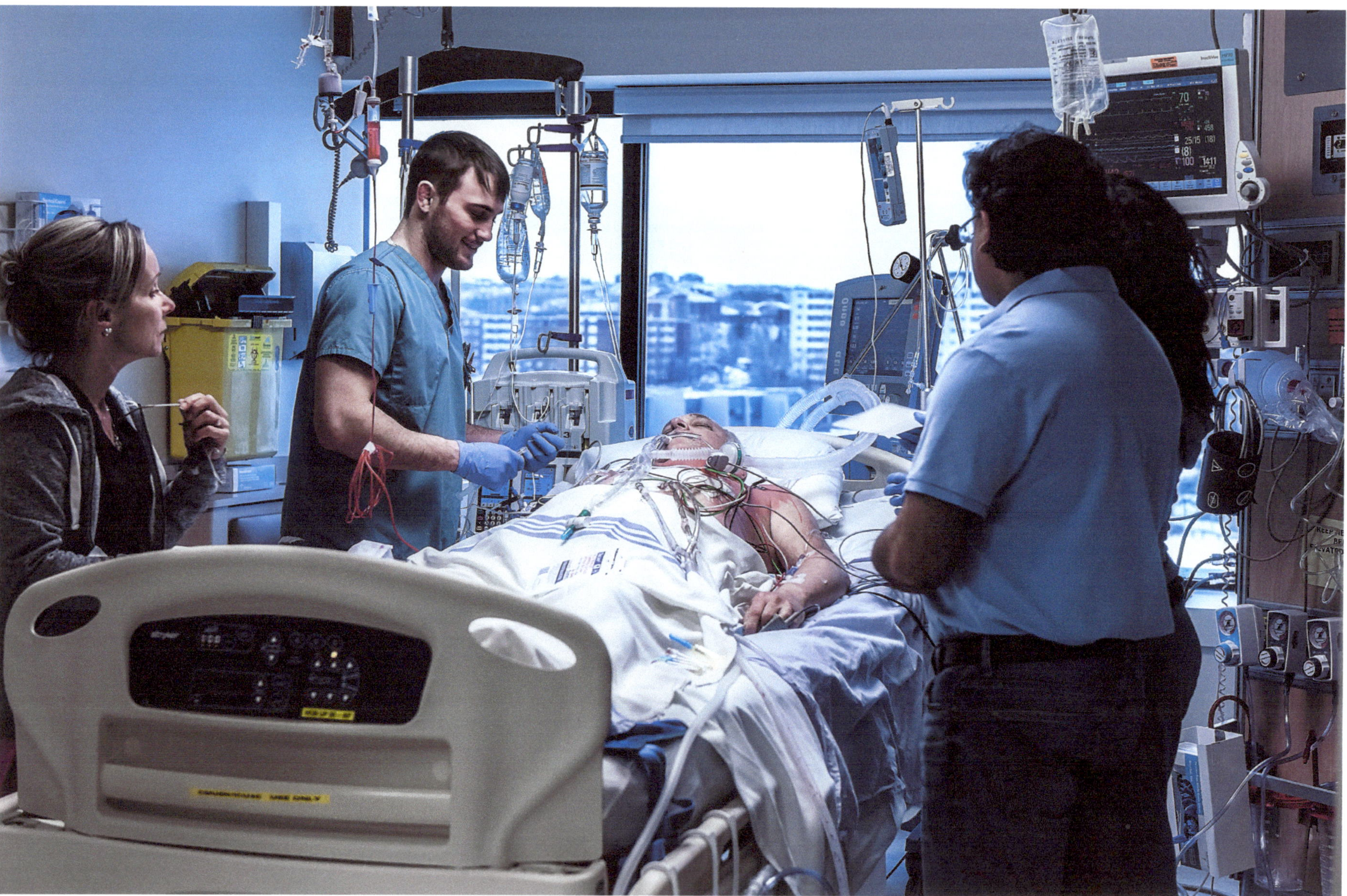

Dr. Garg visiting patient in ICU one hour after surgery

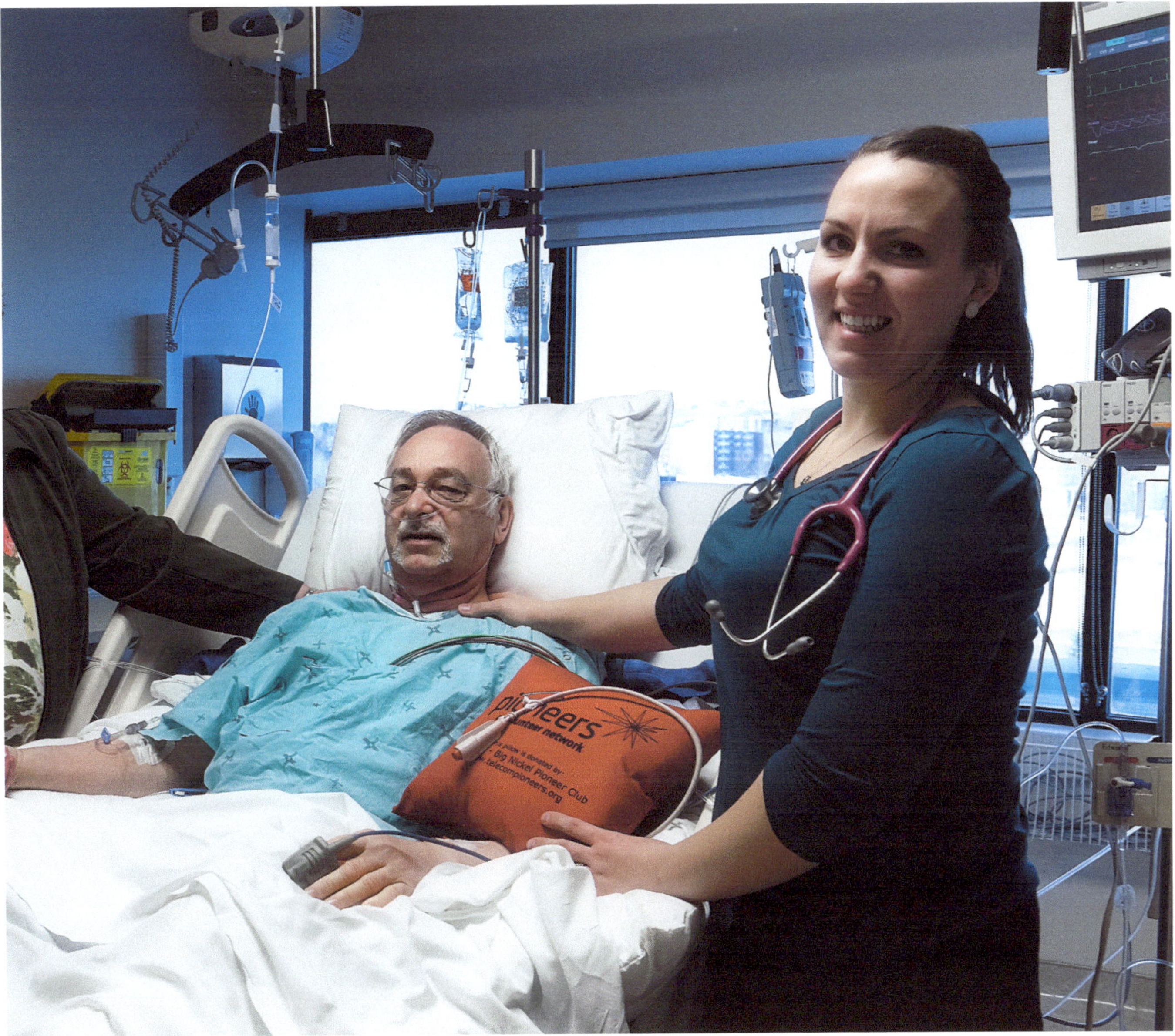

Patient recovering well in ICU twenty-four hours following surgery, with ICU nurse

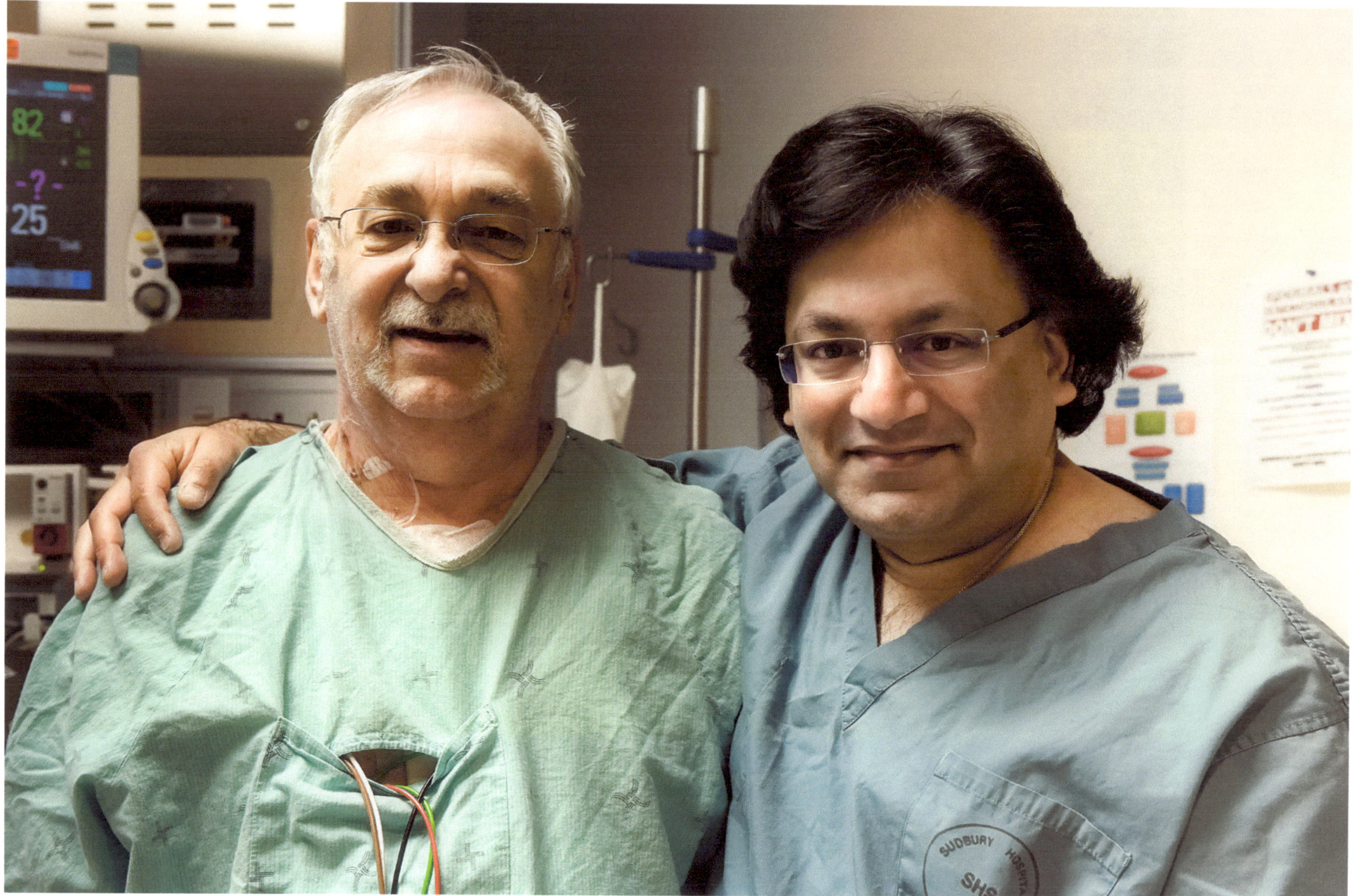

Patient in intensive care unit twenty-four hours following surgery, with Dr. Garg

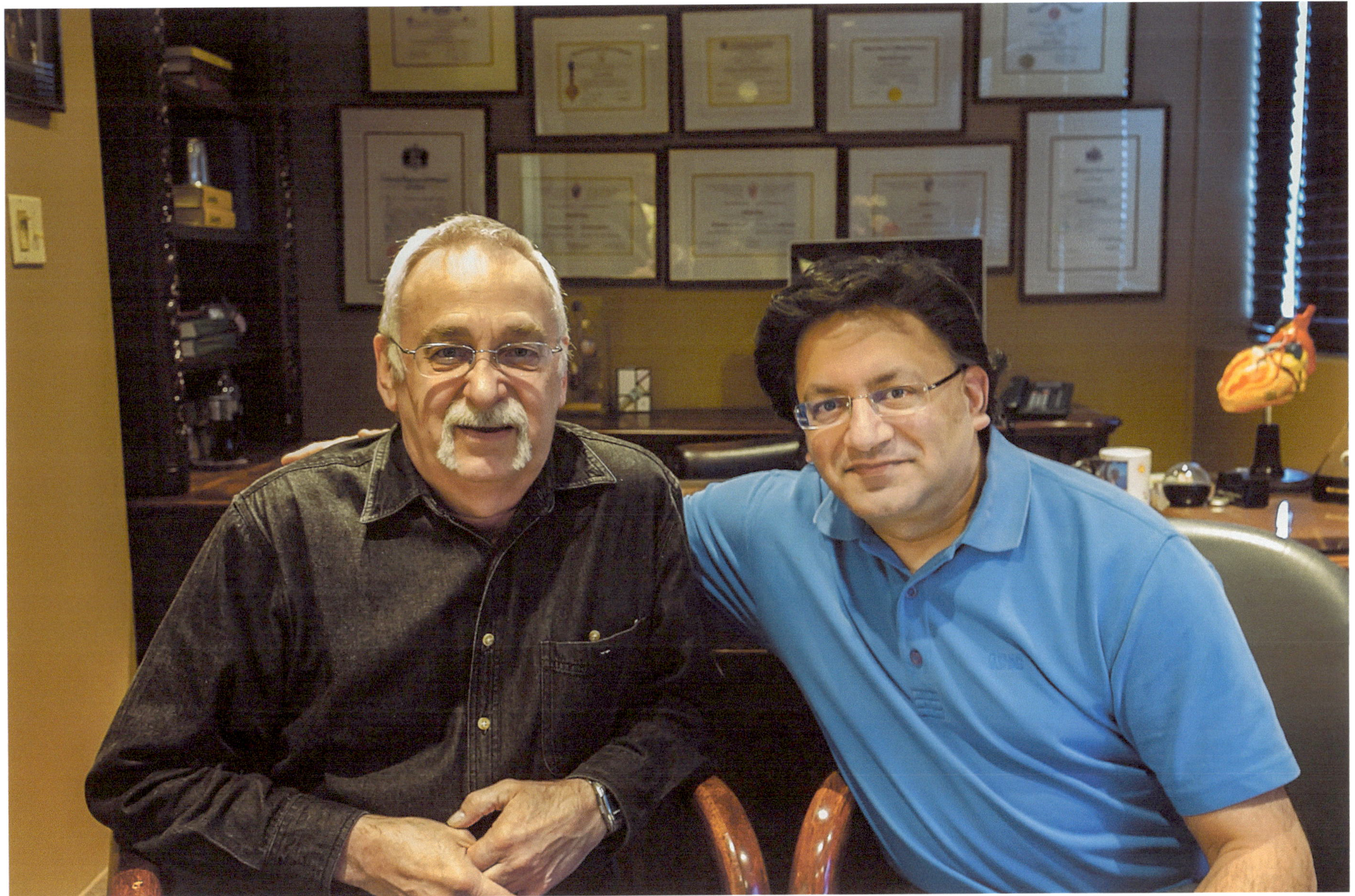

Patient with Dr. Garg at his office—at three-month follow-up visit

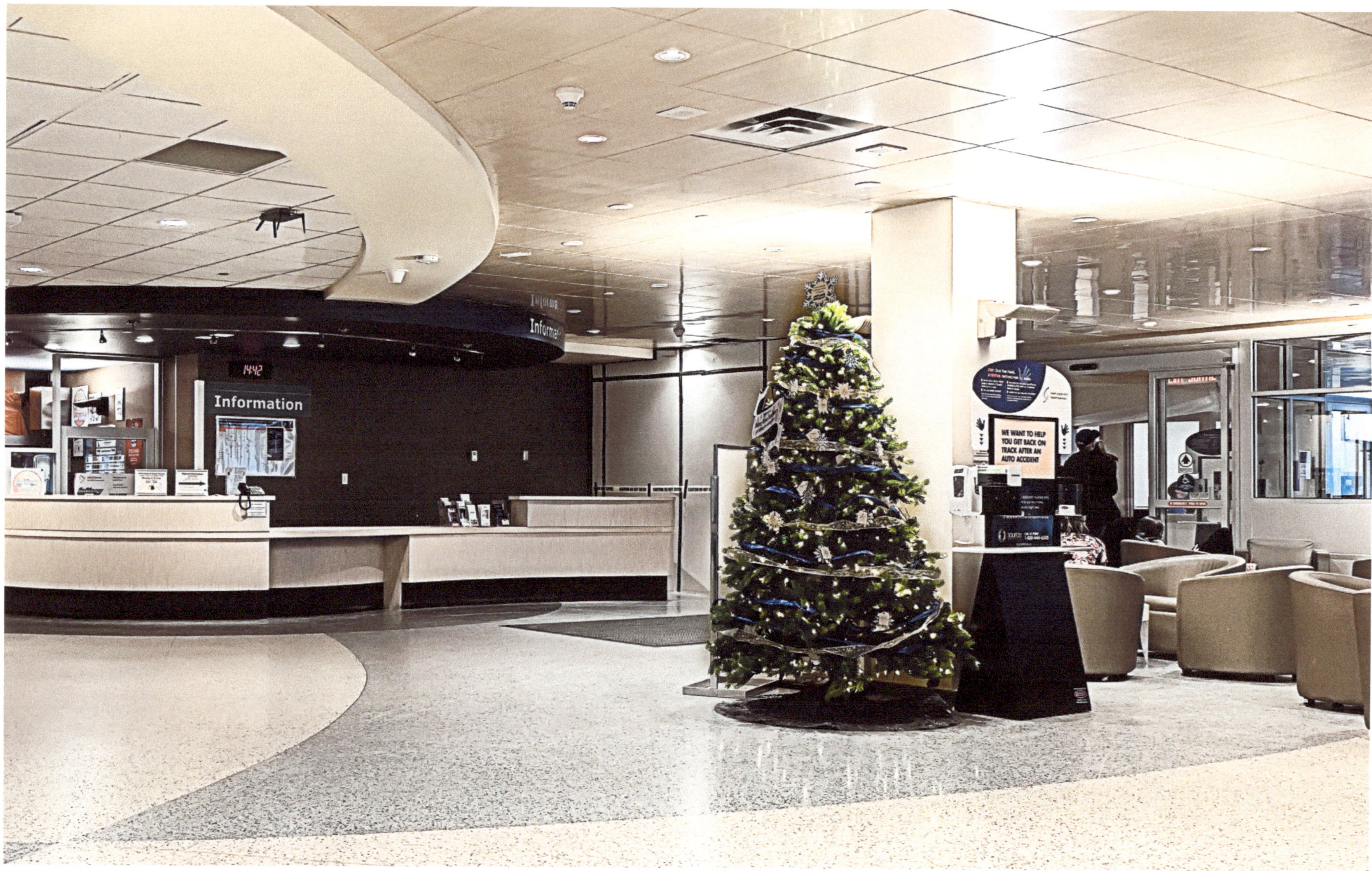

Hospital lobby at Health Sciences North, Sudbury, Ontario, Canada

Acknowledgements

My sincere thanks to management and staff at Health Sciences North, Sudbury, Ontario, Canada, for helping make this project possible.

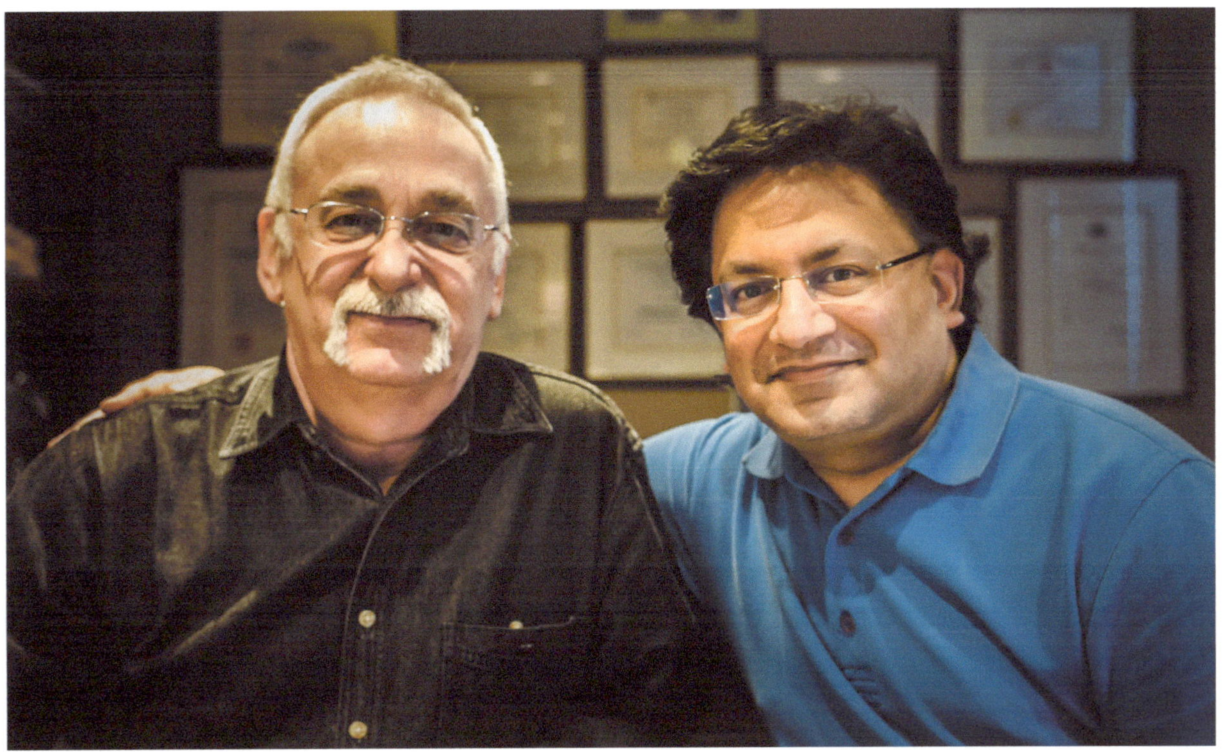

My deepest and sincere gratitude to the patient, Mr. Bergeron.
And, to Dr. Garg, for allowing me into his operating room to photograph the procedure.
Thank you.

MEET THE TEAM

Lead Cardiac Surgeon

Dr. Avinash Garg, MD, FRCSC (*General Surgery*)**, FRCSC** (*Cardiothoracic Surgery*)**, FCCP, FACS**

Raised in Ottawa, Ontario, Canada, Dr. Garg graduated with a Cum Laude Doctorate in Medicine from the University of Ottawa Medical School after attending two years of a four-year Bachelor of Science program from Queens University at Kingston, Ontario. Following a comprehensive Surgical Internship from the University of Toronto, he continued training in General Surgery at the University of Western Ontario, London, Ontario, to become a Fellow of the Royal College of Physicians and Surgeons of Canada. With a keen interest in Cardiac Surgery, he continued with further surgical training in Cardiothoracic Surgery, also at the University of Western Ontario. He received his second fellowship in Cardiac and Thoracic Surgery to become a Fellow of the Royal College of Physicians and Surgeons of Canada in Cardiothoracic Surgery. He then obtained a Fellowship in Cardiopulmonary Transplantation.

In addition to his Canadian fellowships, Dr. Garg is a Fellow of the American College of Surgeons and a Fellow of the American College of Chest Physicians. He is a member of the Society of Thoracic Surgeons, Canadian Cardiovascular Society, and the Canadian Society of Cardiac Surgeons. He is an Active staff and Chief of Cardiac Surgery at Health Sciences North. He has been in cardiac surgical practice for over twenty years.

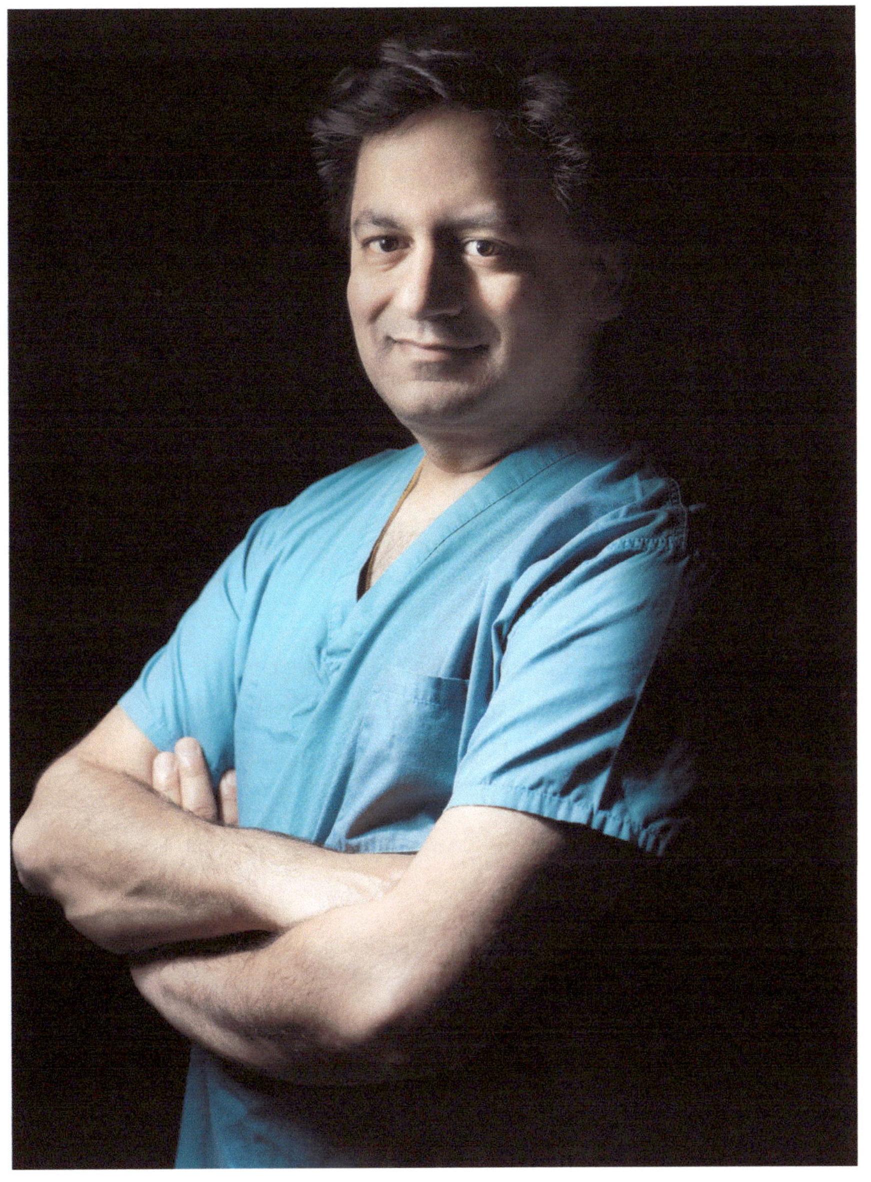

Cardiac Surgeon, Avinash Garg MD

Anesthesiologist

Dr. Jeremie Stewart, MD, FRCPC

Dr Stewart is an Active staff anesthesiologist at Health Sciences North, also serving as an Assistant Professor at the Northern Ontario School of Medicine in Sudbury, Ontario, Canada. Following his Bachelor of Science from Laurentian University in Sudbury, he received his medical degree from the University of Ottawa. He continued with further training in Anesthesia, also at the University of Ottawa, and went on to continue his training in Cardiac Anesthesiology at the Ottawa Heart Institute. He is a Fellow of the Royal College of Physicians and Surgeons of Canada. He is a member of the Canadian Anesthesiologists' Society and the Society of Cardiovascular Anesthesiologists.

First Assistant

Dr. Rony Atoui, MD, MSc, FRCSC, FACS

Dr Atoui is an Active staff cardiac surgeon at Health Sciences North, also serving as an Assistant Professor at the Northern Ontario School of Medicine in Sudbury, Ontario, Canada. He earned a Bachelor of Science and medical degree from McGill University, where he further acquired training in Cardiac Surgery and also obtained a Masters in Experimental Surgery. He completed a clinical fellowship at Northwestern Memorial Hospital in Chicago. He is a Fellow of the Royal College of Physicians and Surgeons of Canada and a Fellow of the American College of Surgeons. He is a member of the Society of Thoracic Surgeons, American Heart Association, European Association for Cardiothoracic Surgery, International Society for Minimally Invasive Cardiothoracic Surgery, and Canadian Cardiovascular Society.

Second Assistant

Dr. Ting-Bong Chow, MD

Dr. Chow is a General Physician and has been in Family Practice in Sudbury for the last thirty years. He has also been assisting in the operating room for several years.

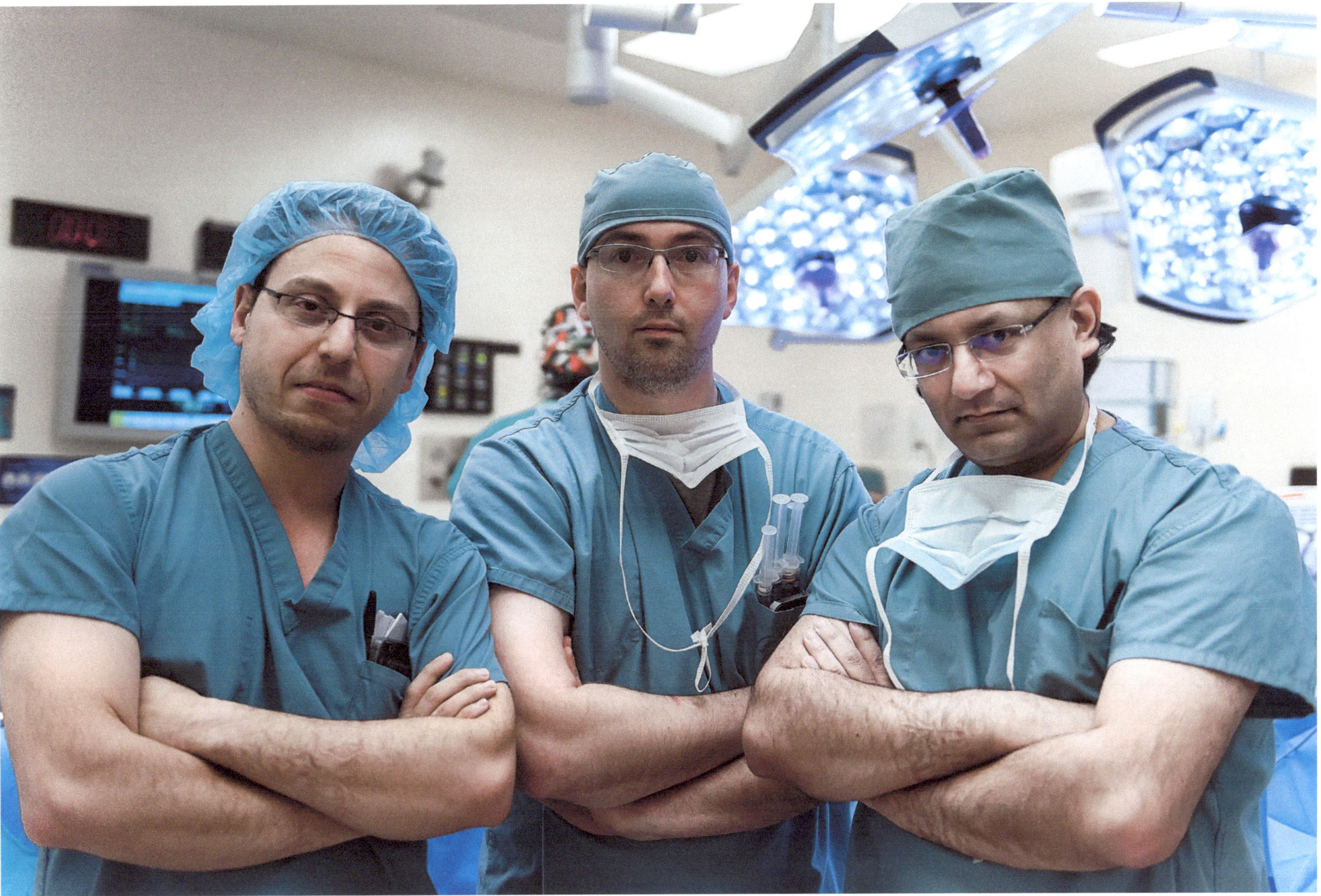

From left to right: Cardiac surgeon, Dr. Rony Atoui; Anesthetist, Dr. Jeremie Stewart; Cardiac Surgeon, Dr. Avinash Garg

Perfusionist

Tova Jessup

Tova Jessup received an Honours Bachelor of Science in Medical Biology from Laurentian University in Sudbury and went on to receive a Masters in Human Health and Nutritional Sciences from the University of Guelph in Guelph, Ontario. She continued with training in Cardiovascular Perfusion at the Michener Institute of Education in Toronto, Ontario. She received the Governor General's Silver Medal Award in Perfusion. She is a board certified Perfusionist, certified by the American Board of Cardiovascular Perfusion as well as the Canadian Society of Cardiovascular Perfusion.

Operating Room Nurse

Louise Doumith

Louise Doumith trained in nursing in Sudbury and is a Registered Nurse. She began her career as an operating room nurse in Louisiana and subsequently in Qatar. She returned to Sudbury in 1980 and has been with Health Sciences North since.

Operating Room Nurse

Chantal Mazzerole

Chantal Mazzerole is a Registered Practical Nurse from Sudbury. She continued with further training as an Operating Room Nurse and has been at Health Sciences North for over fifteen years.

Operating Room Nurse

Petar Valentic

Petar Valentic received his training in Nursing in Slavonski Brod, Croatia. Upon moving to Canada, he received further training and obtained Canadian Certification in Nursing. Petar is a Registered Nurse and has been working in the Operating Room at Health Sciences North for over twenty years.

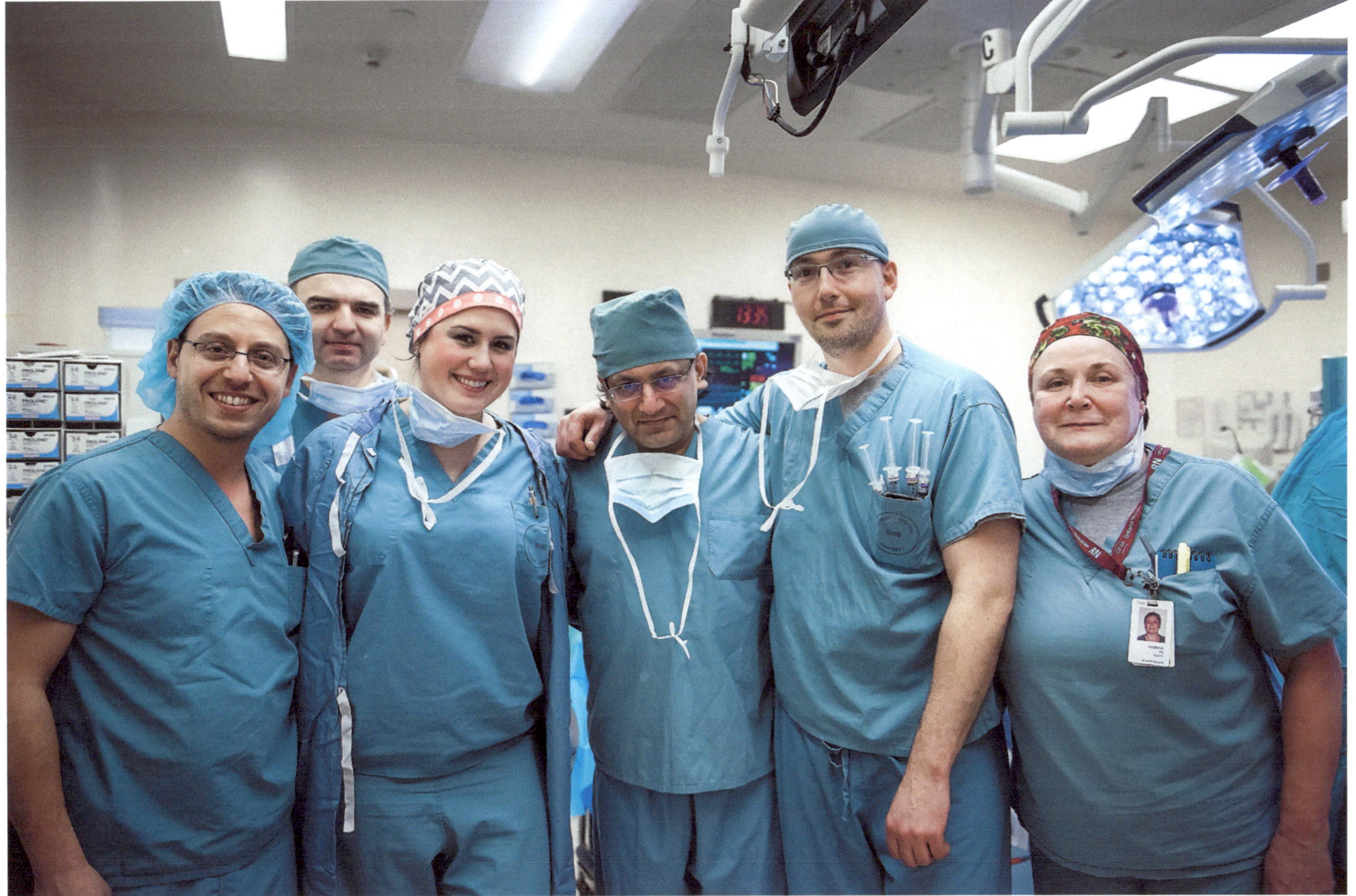

From left to right: Cardiac surgeon, Dr. Rony Atoui; Perfusionist, Tova Jessup; Cardiac Surgeon, Dr. Avinash Garg; Anesthetist, Dr. Jeremie Stewart; Operating Room Nurse, Louise Doumith
Back Row: Operating Room Nurse, Petar Valentic
Not present in photograph: First Assistant, Dr. T. Chow; Operating Room Nurse, Chantal Mazerole; Perfusionist, Lee Prevost; Perfusionist, David White

Proud History of Health Care in the City of Greater Sudbury

Sudbury has always been able to rely on quality health care from as early as 1883, when the first hospital was built by Canadian Pacific Railway crews where Lorne and Elm Street meet today.

Today, our modern one-site acute care hospital with its many programs and services has grown from a long legacy of health care.

Over the years, many dedicated staff, physicians and volunteers have worked hard to maintain the integrity of health care services for the people of northeastern Ontario. Their valuable contributions continue to make a mark today, as patients receive quality care as close to home as possible. Patient care is made better with the use of advanced technology and medical equipment that has been made possible with the support received from the foundations, through the generosity of the community and stakeholders. Community activism has also contributed to important developments in our local health care system, such as the creation of the Regional Cancer Program, the transfer of mental health services into local hands, and construction of the new hospital.

Our community can be proud of the legacy of health care services and look forward to continued excellence in patient care.

History of Cardiac Surgery in Sudbury

Healthcare in Sudbury has an extensive background, with the very first hospital established as early as 1883. Through the years, new hospitals were set up to accommodate the growing needs of the community. By 1950, the Sudbury General Hospital was established, followed by the Sudbury Memorial Hospital in 1956. Almost two decades later, in 1975, the Laurentian Hospital commenced offering health services.

The history of Cardiac Surgery in Sudbury is an illustrious one. Dr. George Rutherford Walker, a General and Thoracic surgeon, began his practice in Sudbury in 1949, following his surgical training in Toronto. Before beginning his practice, Dr. Walker served as a surgeon in the Royal Canadian Navy during the Second World War. In 1955, Dr. Paul Field arrived in Sudbury to work as a surgical assistant to Dr. Walker, who encouraged Dr. Field to continue with his surgical training. From 1957, Dr. Field received further training in Toronto, in England with Dr. Ronald Belsey, a renowned thoracic surgeon and in Boston under Dr. Robert. R. Linton, a renowned vascular surgeon. He returned to Sudbury in 1962 and began cardiac and vascular research in 1963, and by 1965, he established a full-time laboratory at Laurentian University in Sudbury. At the same time in 1962, Dr. Walker was involved in the planning of a Cardiovascular and Chest Unit at the Memorial Hospital.

In 1965, Dr. Field went to Toronto General Hospital for further cardiovascular surgery training with Dr. Wilfred G. Bigelow, one of the most distinguished and pre-eminent cardiac surgeons of Canada. Upon his return to Sudbury, the Cardiovascular and Chest Unit eventually led to the formation of the Cardiovascular Division at the Memorial Hospital and was the beginning of the Cardiac Surgical Program in Sudbury.

Dr. Field performed Canada's first coronary artery bypass grafting surgery in Sudbury, on December 4, 1968. By 1976, the Ontario Ministry of Health designated Sudbury Memorial Hospital as the Regional Cardiovascular Center for Northeastern Ontario. This meant patients from the surrounding area could be offered cardiac health services in Sudbury and therefore avoid lengthy travel to larger metropolitan health centers in Ontario. In 1977, the first Intra-aortic balloon pump (IABP) in Canada was used at the Sudbury Memorial Hospital. An IABP is a pump device inserted through the femoral artery to support a failing heart. In the mid-1980s, Dr. Field also uniquely used the cardiopulmonary bypass machine to re-warm and resuscitate a fifteen-year-old boy brought into emergency, frozen and pronounced dead on arrival. The boy survived with full neurological function. Dr. Walker and Dr. Field, with the help of Dr. Bigelow, were founders of Cardiovascular Surgery in Sudbury.

In 2010, all hospitals integrated to the new one-site hospital, Health Sciences North. Expansion and improvements in patient care by way of specialized equipment, teaching, and research is made possible through funding disbursed by the Health Sciences North Foundation. The charitable foundation is the fundraising branch of Health Sciences North dedicated to providing excellence in health care for the community.

Health Sciences North continues the legacy of Dr. Walker and Dr. Field in cardiac surgery and offers comprehensive cardiovascular healthcare to Sudbury and Northeastern Ontario.

Ann Gilchrist

BSEE, MScEE

Artist, Electrical Engineer

Ann Gilchrist's professional background is in engineering with a Bachelor of Science in Electrical Engineering from the University of Houston, Texas, USA, followed by a Masters of Science in Electrical Engineering from the University of Western Ontario, London, Ontario, Canada. With a penchant for fine art from an early age, her interests quickly drifted from engineering towards art. Following a course in representational art at the Academy of Realist Art in Toronto, Canada and better equipped with formal technique, she began doing portraiture and landscapes in charcoal, pastels and oils. An interest that essentially began as a hobby, turned into a passion in short order. To explore further, she needed her own source material which led her to photography, a vast subject in itself. The camera's ability to capture the play of light and shadows is alluring. Today, photography has also become a major avenue for her visual art expression. Professionally, working with Dr. Garg, provided her with a unique insight into cardiac surgery as experienced by patients and their families. She decided to use her background in art and photography to present a photographic essay in cardiac surgery which culminated into this book. Photographs have been taken with a Nikon D810 and a Leica MP 240.